D1447105

Thieme

# Bipolar Affective Disorders

Etiology and Treatment

Jörg Walden
Heinz Grunze

12 figures
27 tables

2nd edition

Georg Thieme Verlag
Stuttgart · New York

*Prof. Dr. Dr. Jörg Walden*
Universitätsklinik für Psychiatrie
und Psychosomatik
Abt. für Psychiatrie und Psychotherapie
Universität Freiburg
Hauptstraße 5
79104 Freiburg i. Br.

*Dr. Heinz Grunze*
Psychiatrische Universitäts-Klinik
Ludwig-Maximilians-Universität
Nußbaumstraße 7
80336 München

Translation of the German edition:
R. E. Dunmur, Ditzingen

*Bibliografische Information der
Deutschen Bibliothek*

Die Deutsche Bibliothek verzeichnet
diese Publikation in der Deutschen
Nationalbibliografie; detaillierte bibliografische Daten sind im Internet über http://
dnb.ddb.de abrufbar.

© 2004 Georg Thieme Verlag
Rüdigerstraße 14
D-70469 Stuttgart
Homepage: http://www.thieme.de

Printed in Germany

Cover design: Thieme Verlagsgruppe
Cover graphic: Martina Berge, Erbach
Graphics: Ziegler + Müller,
    Kirchentellinsfurt
Typesetting: Ziegler + Müller,
    Kirchentellinsfurt
    System: 3B2 (6.05)
Printing: Grammlich, Pliezhausen
Bookbinding: Held, Rottenburg

ISBN 3-13-1...
ISBN 1-58890-292-7 (TNY)

1 2 3 4 5 6

**Important Note:** Medicine is an ever-changing science undergoing continual development. Research and clinical experience are continually expanding our knowledge, in particular our knowledge of proper treatment and drug therapy. Insofar as this book mentions any dosage or application, readers may rest assured that the authors, editors, and publishers have made every effort to ensure that such references are in accordance with **the state of knowledge at the time of production of the book.**

Nevertheless, this does not involve, imply, or express any guarantee or responsibility on the part of the publishers in respect to any dosage instructions and forms of applications stated in the book. **Every user is requested to examine carefully** the manufacturers' leaflets accompanying each drug and to check, if necessary in consultation with a physician or specialist, whether the dosage schedules mentioned therein or the contraindications stated by the manufacturers differ from the statements made in the present book. Such examination is particularly important with drugs that are either rarely used or have been newly released on the market. Every dosage schedule or every form of application used is entirely at the user's own risk and responsibility. The authors and publishers request every user to report to the publishers any discrepancies or inaccuracies noticed.

# Preface for the 2nd revised edition

Bipolar disorder has increasingly become a main focus of interest in psychiatry. This is reflected by the obvious success of the 1st edition of this book by Walden and Grunze. Due to both the scientific and therapeutic progress it appears now necessary to have this revised version of the book. Concerning therapeutic concepts major progress has been made with the introduction of new antiepileptic drugs such as lamotrigine and atypical antipsychotics to the treatment portfolio of bipolar disorder. But also the scientific evaluation of psychotherapies as cognitive behavioural therapy and psychoeducation constitutes a substantial progress. It becomes clear that modern treatment concepts should integrate both pharmacological and non-pharmacological treatment modalities.

However, despite the rapid increase of knowledge this book is still designed to be a quick reference on the causes and treatment of bipolar disorder, and I hope that it will be a useful tool for the daily clinical practice.

München, Spring 2004     Prof. Dr. H.-J. Möller
                         Director Department of Psychiatry of the
                         Ludwig-Maximilians-Universität
                         München

# Contents

# 1    Introduction

Joseph R. Calabrese

Research on bipolar affective disorder continues to face immense methodological challenges, some of which have only recently become obvious. It has become clear that bipolar affective disorder should be viewed longitudinally rather than in terms of individual episodes. At the same time, achieving adequate methodological rigor in studies designed to evaluate the bimodal prophylactic efficacy has become an important scientific goal. However, due to the illness's inherent complexity, controlled studies have been unable to simultaneously evaluate antidepressant, antimixed, and antimanic prophylactic effects with similar degrees of rigor. Specific, controlled and prospective double-blind studies involving patients who present with mixed states or rapid cycling, as well as patients currently abusing alcohol and/or drugs have previously not been undertaken and only recently have studies on the mood stabilizers been started. But it is just these patients who represent the problem group for clinical therapy.

As a result of these methodological challenges, there have been far fewer mood stabilizers approved for use in bipolar disorder than, for example, antipsychotic agents in schizophrenia, both in the U.S.A. and worldwide. Only 8 years ago, and after a 24-year lapse, did the United States Food & Drug Administration approve a second (valproic acid, 1995) and third (olanzapine, 2000) drug indicated for use in bipolar disorder. In Germany olanzapine was approved in 2002 while lamotrigine, risperidone and quetiapine were launched in 2003. Although this limitation does not prohibit the general practitioner from using alternative, off-label treatments, it significantly distinguishes the pharmacotherapy of bipolar disorder from that of other serious mental illnesses with similar lifetime prevalence. Unfortunately, our patients have probably experienced significant morbidity and even mortality as a result of this avoidance of unapproved drugs.

At present, there are few controlled studies employing greater than 12-month study durations to evaluate the prophylactic efficacy of treatment strategies in bipolar disorder. Nevertheless, there is consensus that there are as yet no certain strategies for maintenance therapy and prophylaxis which result in marked or complete bimodal remissions of new episodes over extended periods of time.

Another aspect undergoing reconsideration is the definition of a "symptom-free" interval. Sub-syndromal breakthroughs and, particularly, short periods of mild hypomania (Keller et al. 1992) have been observed to predict relapse with high degrees of certainty and to have a decisive influence on the long-term prognosis. Accordingly, there is less tolerance for mild sub-syndromal breakthroughs of hypomania and, to a lesser extent, mild depressions.

Lithium, the gold standard of treatment for bipolar disorder over the years, now appears to have a more limited spectrum of efficacy. Recently, the first placebo-controlled lithium maintenance treatment trials were published after almost one-quarter of a century without any studies in this area (Bowden et al. 2000; Goodwin et al. 2003). Recently published naturalistic data also suggest that lithium's response rate has declined substantially in the past two decades, with reported non-responder rates varying from 40 to 54% in 1.7 to 4 year follow-up periods. In the to date largest available prospective, long-term lithium clinical outcome study only 23% of all bipolar I patients exhibited no episodes on lithium and this figure decreased further to merely 14% when reporting no sub-syndromal symptoms (Maj et al. 1998).

These relapse rates are due not only to non-response to the pharmacotherapeutic treatment, but also to poor compliance and the less than optimal use of psychotherapy. In an attempt to approach clinical requirements, naturalistic (not double-blind controlled) studies have recently adopted realistic definitions and designs that allow inclusion of the known, more lithium refractory, atypical variants of bipolar disorder such as affective mixed states, rapid cycling, mood incongruent psychotic symptoms and co-morbid substance abuse. The inclusion of these treatment-refractory variants, especially affective mixed states as well as rapid cycling, has certainly contributed substantially to the apparent deterioration of lithium's response rate. Small placebo-controlled studies have indeed shown that these subtypes predict a poor response to lithium (Swann et al. 1997; Dunner and Fieve 1974). The presence of mood incongruent psychotic symptoms during depression or mania or substance abuse still predicts a poor response to many of the currently available forms of therapy, not only lithium.

When combined, these atypical variants of bipolar disorder actually appear to be more common than the typical classical forms of the illness and probably contribute to the high relapse rate. Analogous to the development of broad-spectrum antibiotics, the clinical management of bipolar disorder would markedly profit from the introduction of a single medicament possessing broad-spectrum bimodal efficacy. Unfortunately, even today only few bipolar patients can be effectively treated with the available mood stabilizers as monotherapy. Lithium, carbamazepine, and valproate exhibit moderate to marked antimanic properties but only low or moderate antidepressant effects. Thus, the concomitant administration of other mood stabilizers as well as antidepressants or antipsychotics is common. But this again leads to a situation where bipolar patients are exposed to an increased risk for drug-induced hypomania/mania, antipsychotic-induced depression or rapid cycling.

The acute and prophylactic management of the depressed phase of bipolar disorder poses a unique and challenging problem. Lamotrigine is currently under intense study as a mood stabilizer with an additional antidepressant activity but with, in contrast, an apparently only poor antimanic efficacy (Calabrese 1999a). In small, controlled studies of bipolar depressive patients lithium showed an effect for over 79% of the patients in 8 of the 11 placebo-controlled studies. However, here again methodological problems limit the generalization of these results. In particular, these studies often included unipolar as well as bipolar depressives and employed crossover designs in which the patients received lithium first and then placebo. Lithium's carry-over effects, discontinuation-induced relapses when switched to placebo, and the short duration of lithium therapy make the interpretation of these results difficult.

Although there are about 10 published controlled studies that have evaluated the relative efficacies of conventional, tricyclic antidepressants in bipolar depression, most studies comparing tricyclic antidepressants with lithium lacked placebo controls. The single study that compared lithium, impramine, and placebo in bipolar depression found impramine to be more effective than lithium and placebo (Fieve et al 1968). The prophylactic effect of lithium against subsequent depressive episodes appeared to be lower than that for manic episodes. On the whole, the interpretation of the above data on bipolar disorder is confounded by significant methodological issues. Most notably, all but one study did not have placebo comparisons. They had unacceptably short study durations and did not control rigidly for the concomitant administration of lithium or the anticonvulsants. The recently published lamotrigine study was the first randomized, parallel-group, placebo-controlled trial to evaluate any monotherapy treatment in bipolar I depression (Calabrese et al. 1999). The results demonstrated that lamotrigine has a significant antidepressant efficacy without any increased risk of switching into mania, hypomania, or mixed states. The clinical improvement became evident as early as the third week of treatment.

Another area of substantial controversy involves the ability of conventional antidepressants to cause switching from depression into hypomania/mania and induce rapid cycling. Reported switch rates in bipolar depression range from 0 to 67% in uncontrolled studies, but are substantially lower in controlled trials. Although antidepressants are believed by many to induce rapid cycling, there is only one prospective, placebo-controlled trial demonstrating this (Wehr et al. 1988), In another analysis comparing 120 rapid cyclers with 119 non-rapid cyclers, only 20% of rapid cycling was associated with antidepressant use (Bauer et al. 1994). Interpretation of these data is also complicated by the absence of standardized criteria for reporting drug-induced mania, the frequent lack of reporting of hypomania at all, the relative absence of such studies in bipolar II disorder, and the generally short study durations. When switch rates were evaluated in a placebo-controlled design, 4.6% of patients given placebo switched over during a seven-week study period (Calabrese et al. 1999 b). With regard to a breakthrough deterioration of an actual episode (relapse), there is currently consensus that the majority of patients with bipolar disorder will relapse either due to poor compliance or due to non-response to the pharmacotherapy.

Many patients experience moderate to marked prophylactic responses over several years of follow-up but eventually relapse. In contrast, other patients report marked longitudinal improvement, but continue to experience clinically significant sub-syndromal breakthroughs that have an impact on their quality of life.

Thus, there is a clear need for new mood stabilizers that possess equal efficacy in depression and mania without the risk of inducing a switch. Such agents would make a unique and long-lasting contribution to the pharmacotherapy of bipolar disorder.

In conclusion, there exists a real need for additional treatment strategies (both pharmacotherapeutic and psychotherapeutic) which, when used in combination, result in marked or complete remission over the patient's entire life span.

The authors of this text have provided the reader with an authoritative and broad-based overview of the state of the art regarding the phenomenology of bipolar affective disorder, its epidemiology, and its clinical management.

Cleveland, January 2004          Joseph R. Calabrese, M.D.
                                 Director, Mood Disorder Program
                                 Case Western Reserve University

# 2 Epidemiology and Social Consequences of Bipolar Affective Disorder

## 2.1 The History of Bipolar Disorder

Bipolar affective disorder has been of particular interest to medical research for thousands of years. The rapid and, for the uninitiated, incomprehensible change from manic to depressive moods and vice versa requires an explanation. At the time of Hippocrates the cause was thought to be a dysregulation of the four body fluids, blood, yellow (choler) and black (melancholy) bile, and phlegm. As early as the second century AD, Galen identified the brain as the site of the illness.

In the first century AD, the Greek physician Aretaeus of Cappadocia first described mania as the phenomenological opposite to depression. After his death he was forgotten until 1554 when his two manuscripts "On the Causes and Symptoms of Acute and Chronic Diseases" and "On the Treatment of Acute and Chronic Diseases" were rediscovered. In these works he described mania as an excessive increase of melancholy, he thus established a unified concept of disease.

This "modern" concept was taken up by French scientists before the turn of the 19th century; Jean-Pierre Falret described "la folie circulaire" to characterize the changes between depression, manic excitation, and a healthy interval. At about the same time Jules Baillarger formulated the concept of "folie à double forme" as different manifestation forms of the same disorder in which mania and depression can occur alternately without the necessity for a symptom-free interval in between.

On the basis of the unified concept of psychiatry proposed by Kraepelin at the beginning of the 20th century, the then used term manic-depressive psychosis included many affective illnesses that are now recognized in modern classification systems as individual clinical entities. At that time Kraepelin still assumed a uniform "manic-depressive insanity" in which, however, he did discuss the important condition, classified today as "mixed states", i.e., the simultaneous occurrence of manic and depressive symptoms. According to Kraepelin, manias and depressions were different presentations of one and the same disorder. Thus, he did not differentiate between unipolar and bipolar affective disorders. The later work of Leonhard led to the formulation of the distinction between bipolar and unipolar affective illness that is still valid today. Among the manic-depressive diseases, Leonhard placed special emphasis on the "cycloid psychoses" that would today rather be classified by modern reductive systems as mixed states. In contrast to the classification system used mainly in the USA – the "Diagnostic and Statistical Manual of Mental Disorders" (DSM IV, Sass et al. 1966) (see Tables 3.**4**, 3.**5**, 3.**6**) to which the classification criteria used in this book refer – the currently valid version of the "International Classification of Mental and Behavioural Disorders" (ICD-10) finally also differentiates monopolar mania more clearly from bipolar disorder. However, studies on disease course have shown that monopolar mania practically does not exist. As a result of more meticulous course observations and the increasing knowledge about the causes of the illness, bipolar disorder is increasingly being subject to a more differentiated consideration. Differences in the prognosis and treatment of the entire spectrum of bipolar disorder are now being seen more exactly for the first time and their special features will certainly be more emphasized in future classification systems.

## 2.2   The Frequency of Bipolar Disorder

The entire spectrum of bipolar disorder according to DSM IV is characterized by the occurrence of at least one manic or hypomanic mood state. According to investigations by Angst (1980) the numerical distribution of recurrent affective disorder amounts to about two-thirds as monopolar depression and about one-third as bipolar disorder.

The data on prevalence also naturally change with changes and expansions of the classification criteria. It is certain that bipolar disorder is not rare. Bipolar I disorder exhibits a life-time prevalence rate of between 1.0 and 1.6% in different countries, i.e., at least one in one hundred people will suffer from the illness during his/her life time. The relatively small range of the **prevalence rate for bipolar**

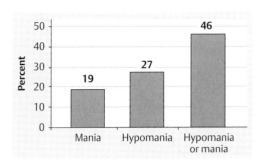

Fig. 2.**1**   Risk for the development of a hypomania or a mania in patients initially diagnosed as "unipolar" (in percent) (Goldberg et al. 2001).

**disorder** compared with that of unipolar depression (between 1.5% in Taiwan and 19% in Beirut, Lebanon) is worthy of note.

The study by Angst (1980) in Zurich came to about the same results. In a later investigation the prevalence rate was found to be appreciably higher (12%) (Angst 2001). Thorough examinations and interviews revealed that many patients initially classified as unipolar depressives had had at least one short hypomanic phase and accordingly had to be characterized as bipolar II patients (see Chapter 3.1). In addition, investigations on the course of patients initially classified as unipolar depressive showed that over a period of 15 years at least one manic or hypomanic phase has occurred in 46% (Goldberg et al. 2001). Since a large proportion of the bipolar patients at first experience depressive phases, they were initially classified as "false unipolar". Thus, it can be assumed that the number of patients with bipolar disorder will rather increase in the future as a consequence of better systematic study designs (Fig. 2.**1**).

## 2.3   Age and Gender Distribution

Bipolar disorder mostly occurs appreciably earlier than unipolar depression, on average about 6 years earlier. 75% of the patients experience their first episode of the illness prior to the age of 25 years as compared to only 55% for unipolar depression (see Table 2.**1**). Among bipolar illnesses, however, there is no difference between bipolar I and bipolar II (see Chapter 3.1).

In contrast to unipolar depression, which affects women twice as often as men, the **gender distribution** of bipolar disorder is about equal. Rapid cycling, however, is an exception (see Chapter 3.5)

Table 2.**1**   Age and gender distribution of depressive disorders

| Unipolar Depression | Bipolar Disorder |
|---|---|
| Worldwide prevalence: 1.5 – 19 % | Worldwide prevalence: 0.3 – 1.6 % |
| Average age at first manifestation: > 30 years | Average age at first manifestation: < 30 years |
| Women affected twice as often as men | Men and women equally affected |

and affects women twice as often as men. There are indications for a slightly earlier first manifestation in women (see Table 2.**1**). However, this may also be an effect of the high co-morbidity with other psychiatric diseases that show a preference for the male sex so that the affective disorder remains initially in the background or is attributed as a symptom of the secondary illness. The natural course of the illness is highly variable. 10 to 15 % of the afflicted persons experience more than 10 episodes in the course of their lives.

## 2.4   Co-Morbidity of Bipolar Disorder with Other Illnesses

West and coworkers (1996) found a **co-morbidity** with other diseases in 86 % of adolescents with a manic syndrome, of these 69 % had an attention deficit hyperactivity syndrome (ADHD), 39 % drug or alcohol abuse, 31 % anxiety disorder, and 8 % Gilles de la Tourette syndrome. The co-morbidity rate in adults at the time of the first manifestation with hospitalization was lower: 39 % of these patients have a further psychiatric diagnosis and 22 % a somatic secondary diagnosis. Again alcohol/drug abuse accounted for about two-thirds of the psychiatric secondary diagnoses.

## 2.5   The Burdens of the Illness

With its relatively high incidence rates, bipolar disorder constitutes a considerable health problem not only for the individual patient and his/her family but also for the economy. Individual patients are in danger of **suicidal acts**, especially in the depressive phase and with mixed mania which, in its mild form, i.e., with less depressive features, is also known as "dysphoric mania". In studies of this affective mixed state by Strakowski et al. (1996) 26 %, or even 55 % in an-

other study, of the patients were judged to be in acute danger of suicide. About 25 – 50% of all bipolar patients make at least one attempt
at suicide in the course of their illness. In this respect, women are affected more frequently than men. During the ten-year observation
period of a Scottish study, the suicide rate in patients with bipolar
disorder was 23fold higher than that of the general population;
most of the suicides occurred relatively early in the illness, namely
between the second and fifth year after diagnosis. A particular, additional risk factor was living alone or in separation; also most suicide
victims came from the lower social classes. This has not inconsid-
erable social-political implications against the background that di-
vorces among bipolar patients are three times more frequent than
in the general population and that the manifestation of bipolar disorder is not coupled to any particular social class. On the contrary, on
average families of bipolar patients have higher educational and in-
come levels than the families of unipolar depressive patients.

The **social-economic consequences** of bipolar disorder have been
investigated most intensively in the USA. In 1985 25.4 million US
citizens aged between 18 and 64 years suffered from affective disorder, 10.8 million of these experienced a manic episode. For the economy this represented a loss of US $ 20.8 billion. This trend increased
in the following years and the enormous sum of US $ 45 billion was
calculated in 1991. In another study (Begley 2001), solely the direct
and indirect subsequent costs for bipolar patients in USA with first
manifestation in1998 were estimated to be US $ 24 billion.

The size of the indirect costs is due, among others, to the large
number of lost working days and early retirements. A German census indicates that the average age of retirement for female bipolar
patients is 46 years and that for male bipolar patients is 46.8 years
(Pfäfflin and May 2002).

The consequences with regard to the quality of life for the individual patient are illustrated by the following estimate from the
US Department of Health, Education and Welfare (DHEW 1979):

A woman who is affected by bipolar disorder at the age of 25 years
(which corresponds to the average age)
- has her life expectancy shortened by 9 years,
- loses 12 years of normal, healthy life, and
- loses 14 years of normal professional and family life.

# 3 Classification and Course of Bipolar Affective Disorder

## 3.1 Characteristics of Bipolar Disorder

Since the work of Leonhard there is consensus that bipolar disorder should be separated from unipolar depression. This is above all of clinical relevance since patients with a depressive episode in the course of a bipolar disorder require a modified psychopharmaceutical treatment that takes prophylactic aspects into consideration as well as having an acute antidepressive activity.

Manic or hypomanic episodes are characteristic of bipolar disorder. Manias are episodes in which the patient's mood is elevated to a degree that is inappropriate to the situation; this may involve increased drive, overtalkativeness, grandiose ideas, flight of thoughts, and a reduced need for sleep. Although the elevated mood is highly characteristic for mania, the patient may also be short-tempered, especially when his/her wishes are not respected. The spectrum of mixed states, already described by Kraepelin, starts here with concomitant symptoms of mania and depression.

In many cases, the manic patient does not recognize that he or she is ill and will not accept the need for treatment. This often leads to "escape maneuvers" and family conflicts. Unfortunately, the consequence is that the urgently needed therapy must often be started against the patient's will.

While a possible diagnostic uncertainty is resolved by the first manic episode, in contrast, it cannot be determined at the first occurrence of a depressive phase whether it is a unipolar or a bipolar affective disorder. As already mentioned, on average 46% of the patients with a prior diagnosis of unipolar depression also experience a manic or hypomanic episode within 15 years. Family histories may give an indication of the respective predisposition.

According to DSM IV, the spectrum of bipolar disorder encompasses the occurrence of isolated manic and depressive episodes (bipolar I) as well as recurrent depression with hypomania (bipolar

Table 3.**1**    The bipolar spectrum: occurrence of at least one of the following characteristic episodes:

| | |
|---|---|
| BP ½ | schizo-bipolar |
| BP I | mania |
| BP I ½ | long-lasting hypomanic episode |
| BP II | spontaneous hypomanic episode |
| BP II ½ | cyclothymic disorder with depressive episodes |
| BP III | long-lasting mood fluctuations under stimulant or alcohol abuse |
| BP IV | hyperthymic temperament with depression |

(after Akiskal HS, Pinto O. Psychiatr Clin North Am 1999; 22 [3]: 517 – 534)

II). In addition, there are marginal forms of bipolar disorder that represent sub-syndromal variants of the fully blown illness. Besides cyclothymic disorder, the so-called hyperthymic temperament deserves special mention. Hyperthymic patients are conspicuous by their enormous self-confidence, they are often highly extrovert and talkative. When they experience a depression this is, for example, classified as a pseudounipolar disorder or also bipolar IV disorder (see Table 3.**1**).

## 3.2    Mania

As mentioned above, mania is characterized by typical symptoms in affect, drive, vital disturbances, and thought disorders (see Table 3.**2**).

For the diagnosis of bipolar I disorder the single occurrence of a manic episode is sufficient. In most cases the patients report that a depressive episode has preceded the occurrence of mania. In the case of bipolar disorder there is a tendency that, with increasing duration of the illness, the frequency of episodes increases as the symptom-free intervals between the manic or depressive episodes become shorter (Fig. 3.**1**).

Since, as a rule, the first episode occurs earlier in patients with bipolar disorder than in patients with unipolar depression, the cycle frequency is on the whole also higher in patients with bipolar affective disorder. A cycle of the illness encompasses the period from the

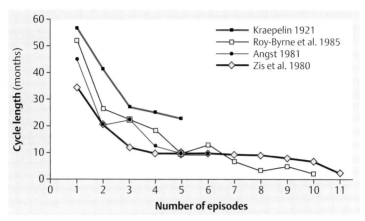

Fig. 3.**1**   Relationship between cycle length and number of episodes.

Table 3.**2**   Symptoms of mania

| | |
|---|---|
| **Affectivity** | Inappropriately elevated mood, sometimes also short-temperedness with aggressiveness, lack of detachment and criticism. |
| **Drive** | There is a strong increase in drive and disinhibition. Often there is a trend for irresponsible buying of expensive objects which can later lead to disastrous consequences. |
| **Vital disturbances** | Reduced need for sleep, increased libido, reduced appetite. |
| **Thought disorders** | Often flight of ideas occurs as a formal disorder of thought (accelerated thinking and jumping from one topic to another) and delusion of grandeur with conceit. |

start of an episode to the start of the next episode, i.e., it includes the symptom-free interval. Unfortunately, a chronic course without intervening full remission develops in up to 14% of the patients with bipolar disorder.

During episodes mood incongruent delusions can occur in about 15% of the patients. Mood incongruence is in distinction to the al-

Table 3.**3** Possibilities for the false diagnosis of bipolar affective disorder as a schizophrenic psychosis

Neglect of the longitudinal course

Incomplete recovery between the episodes is considered as a schizophrenic residue

Equating bizarre behavior with schizophrenic thought disorders

Interpretation of flight of ideas as loose associations

First-degree symptoms are overvalued

most "obligatory" mood congruent or synthymic delusionary contents such as, for example, delusions of poverty in depression or delusions of grandeur in mania. This can lead to diagnostic difficulties, especially when these patients also exhibit auditory hallucinations or other first-degree symptoms of schizophrenia according to Kurt Schneider. However, according to the new diagnostic criteria of DSM IV and ICD-10, all of these signs are still compatible with psychotic mania. The most important diagnostic aid in such cases should thus be the longitudinal course, i.e., the entire previous course of the illness. In addition, bizarre behavior is sometimes psychopathologically equated with schizophrenic thought disorders and flight of ideas misinterpreted as loose associations. An overview of the diagnostic possibilities for mistaking bipolar affective disorder for schizophrenic psychosis is shown in Table 3.**3**.

The diagnostic criteria for a manic episode are listed in Table 3.**4**. Besides these typical courses, many patients (according to recent investigations almost 50%) also have mixed states in which symptoms of mania and depression can co-exist (Table 3.**5**). In the strictest sense, one should only speak of a mixed state (according to DSM IV) when sufficient symptoms are present for the diagnosis of not only mania but also of typical depression. In contrast, the term dysphoric mania is used for mania exhibiting some depressive, mostly irritable, traits but which does not fulfill all of the criteria for a depression. The frequency of such mixed states usually increases with the duration of the illness.

Table 3.**4**   Criteria for a manic episode (according to DSM IV)

**A** A distinct period of abnormally and persistently elevated, expansive or irritable mood, lasting at least one week (or any duration if hospitalization is necessary).

**B** During the period of mood disturbance, three (or at least four in cases of merely irritable mood) of the following have persisted to a significant degree
- inflated self-esteem or grandiosity
- decreased need for sleep (e.g., feels rested after only 3 hours of sleep)
- more talkative than usual or pressure to keep talking
- flight of ideas or subjective experience that thoughts are racing
- distractibility (i.e., attention too easily drawn to unimportant or irrelevant external stimuli)
- increase in goal-directed activity (either socially, at work or school, or sexually) or psychomotor agitation
- excessive involvement in pleasurable activities that have a high potential for painful consequences (e.g., engaging in unrestrained buying sprees, sexual indiscretions, or foolish business investments).

**C** The symptoms do not meet the criteria of a mixed episode.

**D** The affective disorder is sufficiently severe to cause marked impairment in occupational functioning or in usual social activities or relationships with others, or to necessitate hospitalization to prevent harm to self or others, or there are psychotic features.

**E** The symptoms are not due to the direct physiological effects of a substance (e.g., drug of abuse, medication, or other treatment) or a general medical condition (e.g., hyperthyroidism).

**Note:** Mania-like episodes that are clearly caused by somatic antidepressant treatment (e.g., medication, electroconvulsive therapy, light therapy) should not be diagnosed as bipolar I disorder.

Table 3.**5** Criteria for a mixed episode (according to DSM IV)

A The criteria are met both for a manic episode and for a major depressive episode (except for the duration) nearly every day during at least a 1-week period.

B The mood disturbance is sufficiently severe to cause marked impairment in occupational functioning or in usual social activities or relationships with others, or to necessitate hospitalization to prevent harm to self or others, or there are psychotic symptoms.

C The symptoms are not due to the direct physiological effects of a substance (e.g., a drug of abuse, medication, or other treatment), or a general medical condition.

**Note:** Episodes that resemble mixed episodes but which are clearly caused by somatic antidepressant treatment (medication, electroconvulsive therapy, light therapy) should not be attributed to bipolar I disorder.

## 3.3 Hypomania

Patients with bipolar II disorder suffer from recurrent depression with hypomania whereby severe manias do not occur at any time, On the whole, bipolar II disorder should rather be considered as an independent clinical entity and not as an abortive bipolar I disorder. This is reflected in investigations on family history where it is found that the relatives of a patient more frequently suffer from the same manifestation of a bipolar disorder. However, the diagnosis is often difficult to make due to the fact that the patients as well as the relatives cannot always remember the hypomanic episodes because they are usually more discrete and mostly of shorter duration than a fully expressed manic episode. Especially after a depression they are interpreted as a normal "recovery". The false diagnosis of a unipolar depression is thus quite frequent.

Hypomanias are characterized as a milder form of mania with usually shorter duration (see Table 3.**6**). The patient has a slightly elevated mood for several days or a few weeks during which he or she experiences increased physical energy and mental creative power. In addition, the sleeping time is usually shortened. Hypomania is thus a weakened form of mania. In contrast to fully expressed mania, the patient is still able to control his/her behavior in a social-

Table 3.**6**   Criteria for a hypomanic episode (according to DSM IV)

**A** A distinct period of persistently elevated; expansive, or irritable mood, lasting throughout at least 4 days, that is clearly different from the usual, non-depressed mood.

**B** During the period of mood disturbance, at least three (at least four if the mood is only irritable) of the following symptoms have persisted and have been present to a significant degree:
  – inflated self-esteem or grandiosity
  – decreased need for sleep (e.g., feels rested after only 3 hours of sleep)
  – more talkative than usual or pressure to keep talking
  – flight of ideas or subjective experience that thoughts are racing
  – distractibility (i.e., attention too easily drawn to unimportant or irrelevant external stimuli)
  – increase in goal-directed activity (either socially, at work or school, or sexually) or psychomotor agitation
  – excessive involvement in pleasurable activities that have a high potential for painful consequences (e.g., engaging in unrestrained buying sprees, sexual indiscretions, or foolish business investments)

**C** The episode is associated with an unequivocal change in functioning that is uncharacteristic of the person when not symptomatic.

**D** The disturbance in mood and the change in functioning are observable by others.

**E** The mood disturbance is not severe enough to cause marked impairment in social or occupational functioning, or to necessitate hospitalization, and there are no psychotic features.

**F** The symptoms are not due to direct physiological effects of a substance (e.g., a drug of abuse, medication, or other treatment) or a general medical condition.

**Note:** Hypomanic-like episodes that are clearly caused by antidepressant treatment (e.g., medication, electroconvulsive therapy, light therapy) should no count towards the diagnosis of a bipolar II disorder.

ly acceptable manner. The transition to hyperthymic temperament seems to be fluid although, however, the episodic course is decisive for the diagnosis of hypomania. 15% of the patients with initial hypomania, however, can experience fully expressed manic phases in the later course of the illness; this then identifies them as bipolar I patients.

Upon the first occurrence not only of a manic episode but also of a hypomanic episode, an organic cause (e.g., hyperthyroidism, intoxication) must always be excluded as a possible differential diagnosis before the diagnosis of a bipolar disorder can be made.

## 3.4    Bipolar Depression

From their psychopathological appearance, depressive episodes in patients with bipolar disorder (so-called bipolar depression) are very similar to the depressive phase of unipolar depression. Possible symptomatic and case history features for differentiation are shown in Table 3.**7**. In general, however, a depressed mood state with loss of energy and concentration also dominates in bipolar depression. In severe forms psychotic symptoms can also be seen in which nihilistic delusions or delusions of poverty are very common. These delusions are to be classified as mood congruent. In addition,

Table 3.**7**    Bipolar depression vs. unipolar depression (modified from Goodwin and Jamison 1990)

| | |
|---|---|
| Age at first manifestation | BD < UD |
| Women/men | UD > BD |
| More frequent in BD: <br>– loss of energy <br>– increased need of sleep <br>– increased appetite | |
| Family history: <br>– unipolar depression <br>– bipolar disorder <br>– addiction | BD = UD <br>BD > UD <br>BD > UD |
| Chronicity of depression | UD > BD |
| Episodes with psychotic features | BD > UD (women) |
| "Hard suicide attempts" | BD > UD (women) |

disturbances of appetite and sleep occur. In general, sleep and appetite are reduced, however, an increased need for sleep and increased appetite may also be observed. Many bipolar patients with depression have accompanying feelings of anxiety. This can also be expressed as inner tension and restlessness. "Self-healing attempts," perhaps with alcohol or drugs, are not uncommon and complicate the course.

The treatment of bipolar depression is often very difficult (see Chapter 5). Administration of an antidepressant drug without concomitant therapy with mood stabilizers always carries the inherent high risk of a switch to mania; avoidance of the use of an antidepressant, however, may also be accompanied by a higher risk of suicide.

## 3.5    Rapid Cycling

Rapid cycling describes a rapid change of episodes in patients with bipolar affective disorder. The original description comes from Dunner and Fieve who coined the term rapid cycling for the occurrence of at least 4 phases of depression or mania within one year. Here, the number of episodes was counted and not the number of cycles, e.g., the change from a manic to a depressive phase followed by a euthymic interval is considered as two episodes.

**Rapid cycling**
Rapid cycling is a special form of bipolar affective disorder in which at least 4 episodes of a manic, hypomanic, depressive mood or a mixed episode have occurred in the past 12 months. The episodes may change directly into an episode of the opposite polarity or there may be a remission period of at least 2 months between the episodes.

About 15 – 20% of the patients with bipolar affective disorder can fall into this category. Rapid cycling can either be present at the beginning of the disorder or can develop during the course of the illness. With increasing duration of the disease the length of the cycles and symptom-free intervals usually become shorter.

Table 3.**8**    Forms of rapid cycling

| Rapid cycling | Ultra-rapid cycling | Ultra-ultra-rapid cycling |
|---|---|---|
| At least 4 phases/year | Continuous phase changes within days | Continuous phase changes within hours |

This form of bipolar illness occurs in women more frequently than in men (ratio women to men of about 2 : 1) whereas men and women are about equally affected by bipolar disorder. In extreme cases, manic and depressive phases can switch within weeks or days (so-called ultra-rapid cycling) or even within hours (ultra-ultra-rapid cycling) (Table 3.**8**).

In addition, there is a small number of patients who suffer from short, frequently recurring hypomanic episodes (with a duration of about 4 days) without depression; this could represent an analogy to the "recurrent brief depressions" (see Chapter 3.6) in unipolar depression.

## 3.6    Marginal Forms of the Bipolar Spectrum and Delineation to Special Forms of Depression

### 3.6.1  Cyclothymia or Cyclothymic Disorder

This involves a group of patients who exhibit chronic, fluctuating isolated phases of affective disheartedness and phases with hypomanic symptoms. The severity of the individual phases does not fulfill the criteria for bipolar I or bipolar II disorder. For the diagnosis of cyclothymia these mood instabilities must have existed for at least two years. In general, there are no symptom-free intervals of more than 2-months duration in this chronic illness. The prevalence of cyclothymia is assumed to be about 3 – 5 %.

A characteristic feature of cyclothymia is that the long-lasting instability with mild depression and hypomania starts in early adulthood and follows a chronic course. Even so, the mood can also be normal and stable over months. In general, an association with an event in life cannot be determined. The patient usually overcomes the mild depressive phases by an increased expenditure of energy (see Table 3.**9**). The transition to cyclothymic, premorbid tempera-

Table 3.**9** Diagnostic criteria for cyclothymic disorders (according to DSM IV)

**A** For at least 2 years the presence of numerous periods with hypomanic symptoms and numerous periods with depressive symptoms that do not meet criteria for a major depressive episode.

**Note:** In children and adolescents the duration must be at least 1 year

**B** During the above 2-year period (1 year in children and adolescents) the subject has not been without the symptoms in criterion **A** for more than 2 months at a time.

**C** No major depressive episode, manic episode, or mixed episode has occurred during the first 2 years of the disturbance.

**Note:** After the initial 2 years (1 year for children and adolescents) of cyclothymic disorder there may be superimposed manic or mixed episodes in which case a bipolar I disorder can be additionally diagnosed. When there are superimposed episodes of a major depression after the first 2-year period a bipolar II disorder can be additionally diagnosed.

**D** The symptoms in criterion **A** are not better accounted for by a schizoaffective disorder and are not superimposed on schizophrenia, schizophreniform disorder, delusional disorder, or a not otherwise specified psychotic disorder.

**E** The symptoms are not due to the direct physiological effects of a substance (e.g., a drug of abuse, medication) or a general medical condition.

**F** The symptoms cause clinically significant distress or impairment in social, occupational, or other important areas of functioning.

ment is fluid, in the latter state a sub-syndromal hyperactivity alternates with phases of reduced drive and reduced energy. These patients bloom in the hyperactive phases and retreat into themselves during the low energy phases. As a result of the rapid change into phases of hyperactivity, these subjects rarely seek medical help.

### 3.6.2 Hyperthymic Temperament

Hyperthymic temperament is possibly also a sub-syndromal variant of bipolar disorder. The afflicted subjects are highly extrovert, talkative, self-confident, and at times expansive. They often occupy highly respected professional positions. It is clear that a desire and necessity for treatment only arises when they switch from their hyperthymic mood state into a depression (so-called bipolar IV disorder).

### 3.6.3  Recurrent Brief Depression

The so-called recurrent brief depression consists of recurring, short depressive episodes (as a rule not longer than 2 weeks). Frequently 8 or more episodes can occur in 1 year. These short depressions are generally difficult to treat with the usual mood stabilizers or antidepressants. The average duration of an episode amounts to 3 days. About 5% of the population is assumed to suffer from these short-lasting depressions.

Above all, the irregular rhythm and the unpredictability of the depressions are a serious problem for the afflicted subjects. Accordingly, the danger of suicide is particularly high in this group. It is assumed that this is a separate clinical entity and that the recurrent brief depression does not belong directly to the bipolar spectrum.

# 4 Biological Findings in Bipolar Affective Disorder

With the help of modern imaging techniques it has now become possible to demonstrate special features and neuroanatomic correlates of bipolar disorder. Recent genetic studies, at least in defined sub-groups – mostly families and ethnic groups – allow the recognition of possible predisposing factors. Concluding from the mode of action of mood stabilizing agents (mood stabilizers), the emphasis of this chapter is placed on membrane and intracellular transport mechanisms.

Stoll and Severus (1996) analyzed mood stabilizers such as lithium and antiepileptic agents with regard to a common mechanism of action. Their literature search revealed the following common features for the most effective substances:

- Inhibition of postsynaptic signal transduction, mainly via a reduction of intracellular calcium release.
- Suppression of the so-called "kindling," an electrophysiological process and behavior paradigm primarily for epileptic seizures that describes the mechanism of increasing vulnerability in the progression of the illness.

## 4.1 Neuroradiological Findings

### Is there a morphological correlate to bipolar disorder in the brain?

The amygdala/hippocampus – prefrontal cortex – mediodorsal thalamus/ventral pallidum/striatum circuitry plays a crucial role in mood regulation. The amygdala/hippocampus complex modulates the activity of both the prefrontal cortex and the subcortical nuclei. Conversely, it also receives a strong feedback connection from the prefrontal cortex (see Fig. 4.**1**).

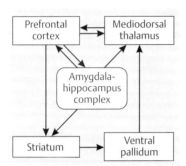

Fig. 4.1  Neuronal circuitry.

Disturbances in the maturation of the individual nuclei of this circuitry or any of the nerve fibers joining them will thus certainly have an effect on the respective other components.

Unfortunately, neuroradiological studies of bipolar patients have not yet produced any unambiguous, reproducible results with regard to illness-typical and illness-specific changes to this circuitry. Not only volume increases but also volume decreases have been described for, among others, the temporal lobes, frontal brain, amygdala/hippocampus complex, and the basal ganglia. Relatively stable and reproducible findings are the MRI signal hyperintensities in bipolar patients, especially in the region of the 3rd ventricle. These appear to correlate with a reduction in the intracellular pH value as measured by $^{31}$P MR spectroscopy. However, since these lesions only develop during the course of the illness they should rather be considered as being of neurodegenerative origin. No indications for characteristic neuronal architecture or migration disorders in the course of the illness which are unique to bipolar patients have as yet been found even in large cohort studies.

On the other hand, the first functional imaging studies have demonstrated a change in the activity of the limbic system of bipolar patients during an episode. Thus, a reduced re-uptake of $^{18}$F-fluorodeoxyglucose by the prefrontal cortex and the left amygdala was observed in manic patients. A PET study with $^{123}$I-iodofetamine of patients with rapid cycling revealed an increased activity in the right, front temporal lobe region during both manic and depressive episodes.

In summary, the first functional imaging studies have shown changes in the limbic system during an episode while MRI provided further indications for neurodegenerative damage in the region of the 3rd ventricle. However, these data must be interpreted with caution since studies on larger patient collectives are still sparse.

## 4.2 Genetic Findings

The relatively uniform prevalence rate of bipolar disorder in different cultural groups, the familial accumulation, and the relatively young age at first manifestation with anticipation, i.e., even earlier first manifestation of the illness in the offspring of inflicted patients, suggest a possibly strong genetic disposition and a lower ability to modulate bipolar disorder by external stressors in comparison to unipolar depression.

Systematic genetic studies are still in their initial phases and the first results are in part contradictory; some reasons for this are related to methodological problems. However, it does now seem clear that bipolar disorder cannot be attributed to a single gene defect but is rather due to the inheritance of an oligogenetic mode. Of particular interest is the concordance rate of 50 to 70 % in monozygotic twins (MacKinnon et al. 1997).

**The search for "hot spots" of bipolar disorder on the chromosomes:** In order to identify genes that may possibly be related to bipolar disorder from the huge amount of human genetic information, the most important starting point is the search for so-called **candidate genes**. These genes code for neurotransmitters or intracellular second messengers that are assumed to be related to bipolar disorder. Examples are the biogenic amines (noradrenaline, dopamine, serotonin) and their downstream G proteins, the GABAergic system, or ion channels (especially calcium and potassium channels). Other potential candidate genes are derived from the sites of action of mood stabilizers such as lithium. The center-point of interest in this search is currently directed at the X chromosome upon which the tyrosine hydroxylase gene is localized and chromosome 18 on which a G protein subunit is coded.

**X chromosome:** Some studies have revealed a co-morbidity of bipolar disorder in families with inherited X-chromosomal diseases such as color blindness, glucose 6-phosphate dehydrogenase deficiency, and factor IX deficiency. A survey of all these studies shows that, at least in some families, X-chromosomal abnormalities represent a risk factor for bipolar disorder although it is certain that there is no monogenetic heredity.

**Chromosome 18:** In a large study involving 22 families, Berrettini and coworkers (1997) investigated 310 autosomal DNA loci, namely chromosomes 1, 5 p, 6, 8, 10 q, 11 q, and 12 – 18 that are under consideration in connection with bipolar disorder. A statistically significant correlation was found between bipolar disorder and changes in the precentric region of chromosome 18 (q11). Among others, a gene for the $\alpha$-subunit of G protein is localized at this site; this gene plays a key role in intracellular transduction and represents a site of

Table 4.**1**    Selected recent results on the relationship between bipolar affective disorder (BAD) and genetic variations of the substances of neurotransmission

| Substrate | Publication | Relationship with BAD |
|---|---|---|
| G-protein $\alpha$-subunit | Berrettini et al. 1994 | relatively high probability |
| Tyrosine hydroxylase | Smyth et al. 1999; Ewald et al. 1994; Kawada et al. 1995 | possible |
| Serotonin transporter | Collier et al. 1996; Kelsoe et al. 1996 | possible |
| Noradrenaline transporter | Stöber et al. 1996 | improbable |
| D1, D2, D3, D4 receptors, dopamine transporter | Cichon et al. 1996; Souery et al. 1996; Kawada et al. 1995; Manki et al. 1996 | improbable; possible for D4 |
| Dopamine decarboxylase | Ewald et al. 1995 | possible |
| Dopamine hydroxylase | Ewald et al. 1994 | possible |
| COMT | Guiterrez et al. 1997 | possible |
| MAO A | Rubinsztein et al. 1996 | possible |
| Potassium channels | Chandy et al. 1998 | possible |

action of lithium. This will be discussed in more detail later. However, it must be mentioned that these studies were not always reproducible and that the clinical response to lithium does not correlate with the presence of this genetic variation. The investigations on other potential gene loci that are decisive for neurotransmitter function also have hitherto not provided any unambiguous results. Worthy of note, however, are studies on positive associations between bipolar disorder and the phospholipase C-gamma 1 isoenzyme and genes for corticotropin-releasing hormone and proencephalin (Turecki et al. 1998; Aida et al. 2000).

Table 4.**1** summarizes some selected recent studies.

## 4.3    Intracellular Signal Transduction and Metabolism

Besides genetics, a major portion of current research is concerned with cellular signaling. Mood stabilizers affect intracellular signal transduction at various levels. These all proceed towards a common final pathway, the **release of calcium** from intracellular stores. The mobilization of calcium not only from intracellular stores but also through influx from the extracellular space is essential for intracellular signal transduction and also for the plastic and functional changes of the cell such as, for example, long-term potentiation (LTP), an electrophysiological model for learning processes.

At the presynaptic nerve endings calcium controls the release of neurotransmitters; it is additionally necessary postsynaptically for the activation of the key enzymes adenylyl cyclase and protein kinase C and thus, ultimately, also for the activation of the so-called early genes in the cell nucleus. These early genes modulate the expression of various enzymes and receptors and so, in turn, again they change the function of the presynaptic side (see Fig. 4.**2**).

The action of calcium is a highly specific and, under physiological conditions, strictly localized process; an impaired intracellular calcium homeostasis on the other hand causes a reinforcement of a number of principally excitation-increasing processes as well as a change in the adaptive, plastic processes in the cell.

A slight increase in the intracellular calcium concentration promotes the cell metabolism. On the other hand, a further increase of the calcium concentration at first dampens the cell metabolism by two mechanisms: blockage of sodium-potassium ATPase (Na/K-ATPase) and adenylyl cyclase. Excessive calcium concentrations in the

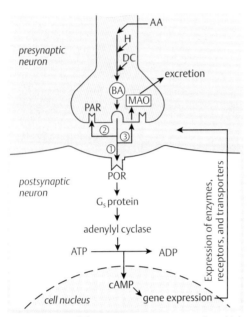

Fig. 4.2   Schematic illustration of the synaptic action of biogenic amines (noradrenaline, dopamine, serotonin). The amino acids (AA) tyrosine or, respectively, tryptophan are metabolized by a hydroxylase (H) and a decarboxylase (DC) to their respective neurotransmitters and stored in vesicles. After release into the synaptic gap, there are, in principle, three possible pathways.

① Activation of the postsynaptic receptor, by which adenylyl cyclase is activated via a G protein and which, in turn, cleaves adenosine triphosphate (ATP) to adenosine diphosphate (ADP) and cyclic adenosine monophosphate (cAMP). cAMP, in turn, diffuses into the cell nucleus and activates the early genes there.

② Activation of the presynaptic autoreceptor by which the further release of the neurotransmitter is prevented.

③ Presynaptic re-uptake of the transmitter which is then either stored in vesicles or is cleaved by monoamine oxidase (MAO) to inactive metabolites which are excreted.

AA: amino acids, H: hydroxylase, DC: decarboxylase, BA: biogenic amines; PAR: presynaptic receptor, MAO: monoamine oxidase.

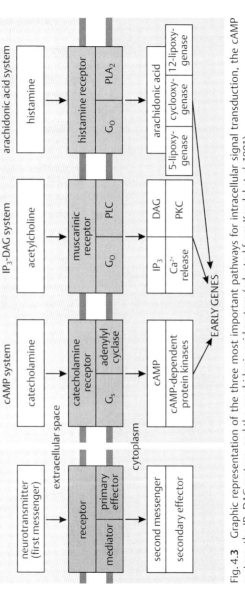

Fig. 4.3 Graphic representation of the three most important pathways for intracellular signal transduction, the cAMP system, the IP₃-DAG system, and the arachidonic acid system (adapted from Kandel et al. 1991).

G: GTP-dependent, activated proteins, s: adenylyl cyclase, stimulating, o: others, PLC: phospholipase C, PLA₂: phospholipase A₂, cAMP: cyclic adenosine monophosphate, IP₃: inositol 1,4,5-triphosphate, DAG: diacylglycerol, PKC: protein kinase C.

cell finally lead to cell death through the activation of calcium-dependent proteases and phospholipase A.

Thus, calcium is on the one hand an essential component whereas in excess it is a cell-toxic component of all three cascade pathways of intracellular signal transduction, namely the cAMP system, the $IP_3$-DAG system, and the arachidonic acid system (see Fig. 4.**3**).

### 4.3.1 Disturbed Calcium Homeostasis and Bipolar Disorder – A Causal Link?

Elevated intracellular calcium concentrations are a stable finding in thrombocytes and lymphocytes of bipolar patients not only under resting conditions but also after mobilization of calcium by means of specific chemical stimulation paradigms. This is valid both during manic and during depressive episodes.

On the assumption that these findings in peripheral cells also reflect the situation in neurons, the following hypothesis, schematically illustrated in Fig. 4.**4**, can be formulated:

■ A slight elevation of the intracellular calcium level activates adenylyl cyclase-dependent metabolic processes. In bipolar patients

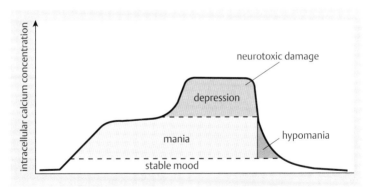

Fig. 4.**4**   Hypothetical relationship between intracellular calcium mobilization and affective episodes. A manic state occurs with a slight increase in the intracellular calcium concentration wheras a larger increase leads to a depressive mood, and an extremely large increase may possibly causes neurotoxic damage. This model also provides a plausible explanation of why many patients pass through a period of hypomania during recovery from a bipolar depression.

this system is possibly already more sensitive to an increase in calcium for genetic reasons. The consequence is, among others, a stronger activation of tyrosine hydroxylase and thus an increased synthesis of excitation-promoting catecholamines. By an additional partial inhibition of Na/K-ATPase and thus a slower repolarization of the neurons the cellular level of excitation increases further; this can be manifested clinically as a manic syndrome. Indeed, a reduced Na/K-ATPase activity has be measured in bipolar patients during an episode of the illness.

- A further elevation of intracellular calcium, in contrast, at first dampens adenylyl cyclase activity to below its physiological level as a sort of self-protection mechanism and can theoretically lead to a permanent depolarization of the cell by a maximal blockade of Na/K-ATPase. The clinical correlate would be the depressive phase.
- During the recovery phase, the decreasing intracellular calcium concentration again passes through a range in which enzyme activity is promoted; this can manifest clinically as a post-depressive hypomanic oscillation, e.g., in bipolar II patients.
- Taken together, this hypothesis combines the particular vulnerability factors of possible genetic origin in bipolar patients such as, for example, altered Na/K-ATPase and adenylyl cyclase activities, with the potentiating affect of an elevated intracellular level of free calcium.

### 4.3.2 Cellular Sites of Action of Mood Stabilizers

How can clinically successful mood stabilizers influence these cellular processes?

**Lithium:** Lithium can act at several sites. It can directly activate Na/K-ATPase and thus partially compensate a reduced activity. In addition, upon activation of Na/K-ATPase, lithium accumulates intracellularly which results in a compensatory outflow of calcium.

The second site of action of lithium is the inositol-phospholipid metabolic pathway ($IP_3$-DAG system) which exhibits an elevated sensitivity in bipolar disorder. Lithium reduces inositol phospholipid degradation and thus the synthesis of inositol 1,4,5-triphosphate which physiologically mobilizes intracellular calcium reservoirs. In this context, Berridge and Irvine (1989) formulated the "inositol depletion hypothesis" which postulates that the therapeutic action of lithium is caused by a reduction of myo-inositol. Furthermore, there are indications that lithium ions can inhibit the high-affinity myo-inositol transport system. Other mood stabilizers such as carbamazepine and valproate may act similarly (Lubrich and van Calker 1999).

In addition, the activity of $Ca^{2+}$-calmodulin kinase II (CAM kinase II) is inhibited. This enzyme is responsible for the persisting changes of synaptic conduction and, among others, plays a role in learning processes.

The other product of inositol phospholipid degradation, diacylglycerol (DAG), activates protein kinase C (PKC). This process is inhibited by lithium. This in turn reduces the synthesis of MARCKS (myristoylated alanine-rich C kinase substrate) which mobilizes intracellular calcium stores and plays an important role for the plasticity of the synaptic and cellular cytoarchitecture. By means of its indirect antagonistic action on the activation of MARCKS and CAM kinase II, lithium thus has a protective effect against structural changes in nerve cells in the course of the illness.

It is interesting to note that the effect of lithium on the $IP_3$/DAG system can thus explain several aspects of the pathophysiology and drug action in bipolar patients.

**Carbamazepine:** Various mechanisms have been discussed for the therapeutic action of carbamazepine such as, for example, blockade of voltage-dependent sodium, potassium, and calcium channels, antagonistic action on glutamate receptors, as well as agonistic effects on GABA receptors and adenosine receptors.

Similar to lithium, carbamazepine reduces the activity of protein kinases A and C via a diminution of cyclic adenosine triphosphate (cAMP)-dependent protein phosphorylation. As a result, the expression of various genes, the products of which are involved in neurotransmitter metabolism, is unspecifically and concomitantly reduced.

However, the decisive mechanism for the antimanic and phase-prophylactic action of carbamazepine may rather be different. Carbamazepine also has strong but, in contrast to lithium, direct, calcium-antagonistic properties. Carbamazepine blocks the so-called L-type calcium channels and thus prevents an excessive influx of calcium from the extracellular space.

**Valproate:** Similar mechanisms of action also appear to operate for valproate, namely blockade of voltage-dependent sodium channels, reinforcement of the rapid, repolarizing outflow of potassium (so-called A current), increased availability of GABA and, in addition, a reduction of the serotonin metabolism. Valproate exerts calcium-antagonistic effects through a blockade of the so-called T-type calcium channels.

Recent investigations have uncovered a common site of action for all of the three mood stabilizers lithium, carbamazepine, and valproate. All three substances stimulate the growth cones of sensory nerve cells. This effect can be reversed by inositol, which implies an activity via inositol phosphatase for all three mood stabilizers (Williams et al. 2002).

**Lamotrigine and gabapentin:** The antiepileptic agents lamotrigine and, to a lesser degree, gabapentin represent new alternatives for the treatment of bipolar disorder. Similar to the other mood stabilizers, both exhibit calcium-antagonistic properties while lamotrigine, similar to valproate, in addition reinforces the rapid, repolarizing potassium outflow.

In summary, all clinically active substances have an indirect or direct calcium antagonism in common (see Table 4.**2**). Thus, it is not surprising that other known calcium antagonists such as verapamil, diltiazem and, especially, nimodipine have also demonstrated efficacy in first open studies on the acute treatment of bipolar patients.

## 4.4 Sensitization and Kindling – Behavioral Models for Bipolar Disorder?

In recent years experimental behavior research has developed several study paradigms that reflect aspects of depression in animal experiments. However, the design of an animal model that also contains the characteristic aspects of bipolar disorder, namely the opposing mood deflections, the changing of symptoms, and the increasing vulnerability with duration of the illness is difficult.

Kraepelin had already noted that the first manifestation of the illness is usually preceded by an appreciable psychosocial stressor and that the significance of the triggering event decreases more and more for the following episodes. At present, these aspects can

Table 4.**2**   Mood stabilizers and their mechanisms of action

| Substance | Clinical efficacy in mania | Clinical efficacy in prophylaxis | Mechanism of action |
|---|---|---|---|
| Lithium | ++ | ++ | Reinforcement of Na/K-ATPase activity, reduction of $IP_3$ synthesis, reduction of intracellular calcium release |
| Carbamazepine | ++ | ++ | Blockade of voltage-dependent sodium, potassium and calcium L-type channels; GABAergic, adenosinergic, and glutamate antagonistic properties |
| Valproate | ++ | + | Reinforcement of repolarizing potassium outflow, blockade of voltage-dependent sodium and calcium T-type channels, indirect GABAergic and serotonergic properties |
| Lamotrigine | + | ++ | Reinforcement of repolarizing potassium outflow, blockade of voltage-dependent sodium and calcium channels, reduction of glutamate release |
| Gabapentin | + | +? | Blockade of L-type calcium channels, possible blockade of sodium channels and indirect GABAergic properties |
| Nimodipine | + | +? | Blockade of L-type calcium channels |

++ efficacy demonstrated in double-blind studies.
+   efficacy demonstrated in open studies.
+? efficacy demonstrated in individual case reports.

best be explained by the phenomena of cocaine-induced behavioral sensitization (CIBS) and kindling as described by Post and coworkers (1995).

### 4.4.1 CIBS – A Model for the Shift of Symptoms During the Course of Bipolar Disorder?

Cocaine causes neurohormonal changes similar to those resulting from stress, for example, elevation of the neuropeptides CRF and ACTH, cortisol, cytokines, as well as catecholamines and indolamine. The acute administration of cocaine results in motor hyperactivity in rats as well as hypomanic symptoms in humans. The repeated administration of cocaine increases motor activity in rats not only with regard to time of onset but also severity. In humans the symptoms are reinforced and shifted towards a marked dysphoric irritability or even paranoid behavior.

Neuroanatomic studies have shown that the repeated administration of cocaine at first leads to morphological changes in the amygdala. The increased behavioral symptoms after repeated cocaine stimulation in the rat, however, occur even after iatrogenic destruction of the amygdala. Apparently other regions of the brain besides the amygdala participate to an increasing extent in the cocaine-induced sensitization model.

The fact that the symptoms can also be reinforced by conditioned stimuli points in the same direction. Many patients report about cognitive reasoning that could be understood as a conditioning process, for example, the anniversary of the death of a close relative, which acts as a trigger for a depressive phase. In addition, CIBS is a model that shows how repeated episodes of the illness can lead to a shift of the symptoms, for example, in the direction of dysphoric mania.

### 4.4.2 Kindling – A Model for the Increase in Episode Frequency of Bipolar Disorder?

The increasing occurrence of episodes in spite of more moderate external stressors can be explained by the electrophysiological model of kindling that originated from epilepsy research. To kindle means to induce a recurring process of increased neuronal excitability which then proceeds mostly autonomously. Similar to CIBS, here again the amygdala complex plays a central role. In rats, repeated electrical stimulation of the basolateral amygdala lowers the threshold for triggering epileptic seizures and also increases the frequency of spontaneous epileptic activity. At the cellular level this occurs through a reinforcement of the glutaminergic transmission with concomitant weakening of the GABAergic activity.

Goldberg and Harow (1994) showed in a group of patients with the same total number of previous episodes that those who had once experienced a pattern with a rapid cycling of episodes also experienced more episodes in the subsequent, prospective observation period. This may possibly be attributed to a kindling process that had occurred previously.

With reference to the above-mentioned investigations of Stoll and Severus (1996) it would be interesting to determine the degree to which lithium and antiepileptic agents can prevent CIBS and kindling.

As already mentioned, lithium inhibits the activation of MARCKS and CAM kinase II by way of its calcium-antagonistic properties and thus partially prevents the neuroanatomic restructuring set in motion by kindling.

Antikindling effects have also been demonstrated for carbamazepine, lamotrigine and valproate; these effects are presumably also due to their calcium-antagonistic properties. With regard to CIBS, it is worthy of note that the calcium antagonist nimodipine, which has become a therapeutic alternative especially for rapid cycling, reduces the cocaine-induced motor hyperactivity in rats.

# 5   Treatment Strategies for Bipolar Disorder

The treatment of bipolar disorder can be divided into three stages:
- **Acute treatment** of an episode of the disorder,
- **Continuation treatment** (stabilization phase) after the acute symptoms have subsided,
- **Maintenance treatment** (episode prophylaxis).

The treatment strategies for the individual phases are complementary and overlap. With regard to acute episodes, again neither mania nor depression is uniform but can rather exhibit various combinations of symptoms. In addition, the best possible tailored acute treatment must not only take the actual mood deflection into account but also the frequency, rapid cycling for example, and the nature of preceding episodes, e.g., manic or merely hypomanic phases. Thus, a drug that is otherwise very effective, such as lithium for example, is of only limited use in cases of rapid cycling.

It is also clear that polypharmacotherapy instead of monotherapy is rather the rule than the exception for optimal treatment of bipolar disorder (see Chapter 5.3.6).

In order to provide the treating physician with rational guidelines in decision making on the basis of experience and studies, expert commissions have developed recommendations for the individual treatment modalities (see Frances et al. 1996, Walden et al. 1999, Grunze et al. 2002, 2002 a, 2003). The indications for the individual mood stabilizers are given in Table 5.**1**. Most clinical experience is available for the three substances lithium, valproate and carbamazepine that are also considered by the WHO as being the keystones of treatment. In addition, the atypical antipsychotic agents olanzapine, risperidone and quetiapine have recently been approved in several countries. Table 5.**2** lists further important therapy modalities for the individual mood fluctuations. It must be emphasized that these tables reflect the current state of scientific knowledge which is not always identical with the drug approval

Table 5.**1**   Indications for various mood stabilizers

| Mood stabilizer | Use |
| --- | --- |
| **Lithium (Li)** | – Good efficacy demonstrated by routine use<br>– Euphoric mania<br>– Prophylaxis for classical bipolar I disorder<br>– Cyclothymia, if treatment is needed<br>– Add-on treatment for inadequate response to another mood stabilizer in acute treatment and prophylaxis<br>– Combination therapy with an antidepressant agent for bipolar depression<br>– Augmentation in case of inadequate response to anti-depressive treatment in uni- and bipolar depression<br>– Patients with liver or hematological diseases in whom VPA and CBZ are contraindicated |
| **Valproate (VPA)** | – Good efficacy demonstrated by routine use<br>– All forms of mania: mixed states, euphoric mania, mania with rapid cycling and psychotic mania<br>– To be preferred over Li for euphoric mania when a rapid onset of action is necessary and/or there is no possibility for close monitoring of the serum Li level<br>– Hypomanic states<br>– Cyclothymia, if treatment is required<br>– Combination therapy with an antidepressant agent for bipolar depression<br>– Prophylaxis in rapid cycling patients and for atypical manifestations in which CBZ and OXC are not effective or are contraindicated<br>– Prophylaxis for typical courses in non-responders to Li and CBZ<br>– Add-on treatment for inadequate response to another mood stabilizer in acute therapy and prophylaxis<br>– Patients with co-morbidity: kidney diseases, CNS diseases (especially migraine), functional stomach diseases (e.g., irritable colon), alcohol or drug addiction, anxiety and obsessive-compulsive disorders |

*continuation next page*

Table 5.**1**  Indications for various mood stabilizers  *(continuation)*

| Mood stabilizer | Use |
|---|---|
| **Carbamazepine (CBZ) and Oxcarbazepine (OXC)** | – Good efficacy demonstrated by routine use<br>– All forms of mania when Li and VPA are ineffective or contraindicated<br>– Hypomanic states<br>– Cyclothymia, if treatment is required<br>– Combination therapy with an antidepressive agent for bipolar depression (note: interaction)<br>– Possible augmentative effect on inadequate response to an antidepressive treatment in uni- and bipolar depression<br>– Prophylaxis for an atypical course of bipolar disorder<br>– Prophylaxis for rapid cycling patients for whom VPA is not effective or is contraindicated<br>– Prophylaxis for Li non-responders with typical courses<br>– Add-on treatment for inadequate response to another mood stabilizer in acute treatment or prophylaxis<br>– Patients with co-morbidity: kidney diseases, CNS and peripheral nerve diseases (especially neuralgias), alcohol or drug addiction |
| **Lamotrigine (LTG)** | – Good efficacy demonstrated by routine use<br>– Bipolar depression, for severe forms in combination with an antidepressive agent<br>– Mixed states when VPA alone is not sufficient<br>– Therapy-resistant manias<br>– Cyclothymia, with predominately depressive states, if treatment is required<br>– Prophylaxis for patients who suffer mainly from depressive episodes<br>– Prophylaxis for rapid cycling patients and atypical manifestations for which VPA, CBZ and OXC are not effective or are contraindicated<br>– Augmentative treatment for uni- and bipolar depression |
| **Olanzapine** | – Treatment of acute mania, especially of mixed states that do not respond adequately to VPA, also available as i.m. injection<br>– Maintenance treatment if manic episodes predominate |

*continuation next page*

Table 5.**1**   Indications for various mood stabilizers   *(continuation)*

| Mood stabilizer | Use |
|---|---|
| **Gabapentin** | – Augmentative administration for therapy-resistant mania or bipolar depression, especially when a co-morbidity with addictive or anxiety disorders is present |
| **Topiramate** | – Additional drug for therapy-resistant mania and inadequate prophylaxis, especially when weight gain represents a problem |
| **Clozapine** | *With consideration of the special prescription regulations:*<br>– Therapy-resistant manias and bipolar depression as monotherapy or in combination (but not with CBZ and OXC, not with benzodiazepines, especially lorazepam) |
| **Risperidone** | – Treatment of acute mania<br>– Insufficient maintenance treatment with other mood stabilizers, especially also for breakthrough episodes with strong psychotic features |
| **Quetiapine** | – Treatment of acute mania<br>– Insufficient maintenance treatment with other mood stabilizers, especially also for breakthrough episodes with strong psychotic features |
| **Ziprasidone** | – Treatment of acute mania, if necessary also as i.m. injection! |
| **Aripiprazole** | – Treatment of acute mania |
| **Clonazepam, Lorazepam** | – Short-term additional drug in cases of inadequate mania treatment, especially severe agitation and anxious tension |
| **Nimodipine** | – Additional drug in cases of inadequate mania treatment and prophylaxis for rapid cycling and ultra-rapid cycling patients<br>– Treatment of refractory depression, especially with rapid cycling |

Table 5.**2**    Further treatment options for bipolar disorder

| Further therapy form | Use |
| --- | --- |
| Classical antipsychotics | – Adjuvant treatment for mania or depression with psychotic symptoms |
| Electroconvulsive therapy | – Bipolar depression with psychotic components; treatment resistant bipolar depression and mania |
| Bupropione | – Depressive patients with a high risk of a switch into mania or rapid cycling |
| Selective serotonin re-uptake inhibitors | – Bipolar depression |
| Monoamine oxidase (MAO) inhibitor | – Treatment resistant bipolar depression |
| L-Thyroxine | – Augmentative treatment for bipolar depression and rapid cycling, co-medication with lithium in cases of elevated TSH or hypothyroidism |
| Combination treatment with mood stabilizer and antidepressant | – Bipolar depression without psychotic components |
| Combination treatment with mood stabilizer, antipsychotic agent and antidepressant | – Bipolar depression with psychotic components |

status in any particular country. For details please refer to Chapter 5.4.4.

## 5.1    Drug Treatment Strategies

The detailed clinical use of the common mood stabilizers is discussed in Chapter 3. This chapter is firstly intended to provide help in decision making about the steps of treatment. The treatment algorithms given here, which were developed during a conference of German experts (see Walden et al. 1999, Grunze et al. 2002), correspond in most aspects with international recommendations.

### 5.1.1   Acute Treatment

**Euphoric Mania**

Prior to starting treatment, at least a comprehensive clinical examination should be performed to exclude a severe physical disease or substance abuse as an organic cause of the mania or which may result in a limitation in the choice of drug. In general, mania treatment is carried out under in-patient conditions which, on the one hand, shields the patient from hyperstimulation and, on the other hand, provides the patient with a protective environment during the acute treatment. Since the patients often do not accept that they are ill, in individual cases it can be very difficult to persuade them to voluntarily remain in hospital for treatment. However, on account of the severe social consequences as well as the possible dangers to others, all measures to retain them, including a court order if necessary, should be considered.

**Initiation of treatment:** At the start of the treatment there is often a necessity for rapid sedation with the patient refusing oral administration of drugs. Even though they carry a high risk of strong side effects and/or have only limited causative anti-manic efficacy according to the current state of knowledge, there is still a place for the administration, possibly by the intramuscular route, of classical high and low potent antipsychotic agents or benzodiazepines. The choice of drug or, respectively, combination of drugs depends on the degree of excitation and the possible presence of psychotic symptoms. Administration of short-lasting, depot antipsychotic drugs (e.g., zuclopentixol) may also be considered.

A disadvantage here is, however, the limited control of the drug, for example in cases of strong orthostatic side effects, dyskinesias, allergic reactions or even a malignant neuroleptic syndrome. The rate of tardive dyskinesias through administration of antipsychotic agents in patients with bipolar disease is about three times higher than that in patients with schizophrenic psychoses (Mukherjee et al. 1986). Ziprasidone and olanzapine, atypical antipsychotic agents that can also be administered intramuscularly, exhibit a better profile of side effects, especially with regard to extrapyramidal motor side effects. Open and controlled studies indicate that they have a comparable activity to haloperidol or lorazepam for acute states of excitation.

**Lithium:** For patients who will voluntarily take the prescribed drugs, lithium remains the classical agent for the treatment of acute euphoric mania. In addition, since most patients have previously taken lithium as maintenance treatment so that its tolerability can be estimated, the first rational step is to increase the lithium dose up to serum levels in the upper range. Before such measures are taken, the lithium level should be determined at admission; it is well known that discontinuation of lithium or unreliable consumption of the drug is frequently the reason for a recurrence of the illness. On the other hand, the safety of lithium therapy with rapidly increasing doses is poor; that is why this therapeutic strategy has become increasingly less important in the past few years.

Depending on the type and extent of the symptoms, lithium can and should be given primarily either together with a sedative (benzodiazepines, e.g., clonazepam) or combined with an antipsychotic agent when psychotic symptoms are present. Especially for severe manias, lithium as monotherapy appears to be inferior to the classical antipsychotic agents (Northwick Park Study, Johnstone et al. 1988).

**Lithium doesn't work – what next? The role of antiepileptic agents:** If, in spite of a lithium level in the upper range (> 1 mmol/l), no improvement of the symptoms can be observed after one week, an overlapping therapy attempt with antiepileptic or atypical antipsychotic agents such as, e.g., olanzapine, quetiapine or risperidone, is indicated. Then it must be decided whether lithium is to be continued in a combination therapy or tapered off. A major factor for this is the individual history, whether there was a response to lithium in previous episodes and if a later continuation of lithium as maintenance therapy makes sense. In the latter case, lithium should not be discontinued in order to avoid a possible loss of efficacy of lithium in the prophylaxis.

The available agents of choice, as far as antiepileptic drugs are concerned, are carbamazepine, oxcarbazepine, valproate and, albeit with limitations, clonazepam. Here again, combination with a sedative or an antipsychotic agent is possible and may be necessary. Alternatively, an attempt with the add-on administration of, in particular, an atypical antipsychotic agent may be made. However, special attention must be paid to interactions (e.g., clozapine – carbamazepine: agranulocytosis; clozapine – lorazepam: respiratory arrest;

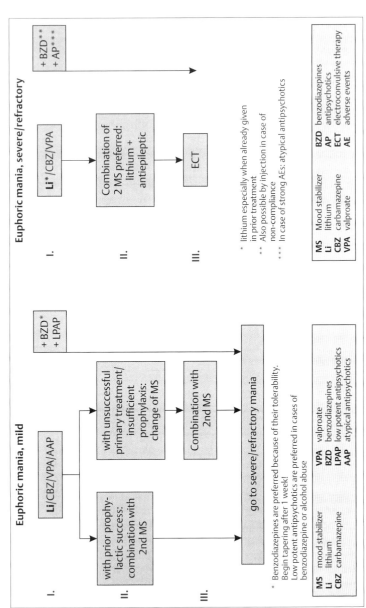

Fig. **5.1**   Treatment algorithm for euphoric mania.

**Euphoric mania, mild**

I.   Li/CBZ/VPA/AAP

II.  with prior prophy-lactic success: combination with 2nd MS

     with unsuccessful primary treatment/ insufficient prophylaxis: change of MS

                    + BZD*
                    + LPAP

     Combination with 2nd MS

III. go to severe/refractory mania

* Benzodiazepines are preferred because of their tolerability. Begin tapering after 1 week!
  Low potent antipsychotics are preferred in cases of benzodiazepine or alcohol abuse

| MS | mood stabilizer | VPA | valproate |
|---|---|---|---|
| Li | lithium | BZD | benzodiazepines |
| CBZ | carbamazepine | LPAP | low potent antipsychotics |
| | | AAP | atypical antipsychotics |

**Euphoric mania, severe/refractory**

I.   Li*/CBZ/VPA

                    + BZD**
                    + AP***

II.  Combination of 2 MS preferred: lithium + antiepileptic

III. ECT

* lithium especially when already given in prior treatment
** Also possible by injection in case of non-compliance
*** In case of strong AEs: atypical antipsychotics

| MS | Mood stabilizer | BZD | benzodiazepines |
|---|---|---|---|
| Li | lithium | AP | antipsychotics |
| CBZ | carbamazepine | ECT | electroconvulsive therapy |
| VPA | valproate | AE | adverse events |

carbamazepine – haloperidol: loss of efficacy due to lowered halo-peridol blood levels; lithium – highly potent antipsychotics: neuro-toxicity).

If these polytherapies are also not successful, a combination with the calcium channel blocker nimodipine or with one of the newer antiepileptics such as levatiracetam may also be tried.

In the particular light of the increasing risk of interactions with polypharmacotherapies, the next step to be considered should be electroconvulsive therapy (ECT, see below).

Fig. 5.**1** summarizes the above considerations as a treatment algorithm for mild to moderate and severe euphoric manias.

**Mixed States and Dysphoric Mania**

The treatment algorithms for a mixed episode and for dysphoric mania are similar except that in these cases valproate and olanzapine are the agents of first choice while carbamazepine and lithium are the second choice. Furthermore, in cases of marked depressive symptoms lasting for more than one week add-on administration of lamotrigine may be considered. If the use of an antidepressant seems to be unavoidable in exceptional cases, tri- and tetracyclic antidepressants must not be used. In a high percentage of patients these agents can, without the concomitant protection of a mood stabilizer, induce an intensification of the manic symptoms. This risk seems to be lower with the selective serotonin re-uptake inhibitors and bupropione – which is only approved in several countries for nicotine withdrawal symptoms. Also, one study has shown that the irreversible MAO A inhibitor tranylcypromine is superior to the reference drug imipramine in treating depressive symptoms in the course of a mixed state. Thus, these three groups of substances should be taken as agents of first choice. In cases of treatment re-fractoriness, ECT should be considered at an early stage, especially because of the danger of suicidal acts.

The treatment algorithm for mixed mania is shown in Fig. 5.**2**.

**Rapid Cycling**

Rapid cycling creates particular treatment problems because lithium exhibits only a low efficacy and appears to be without prophy-lactic effects against depressive episodes. Valproate, olanzapine and

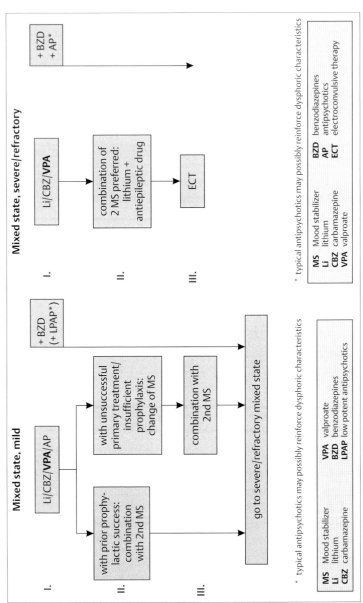

Fig. 5.2   Treatment algorithm for mixed mania.

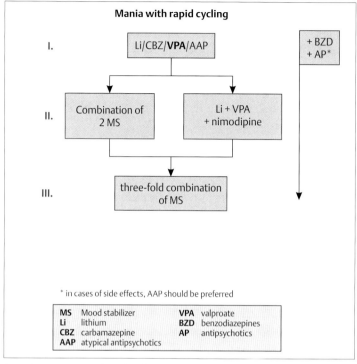

Fig. 5.**3** Treatment algorithm for rapid cycling.

possibly also carbamazepine appear to be superior. Taking long-term prophylactic aspects into account, lamotrigine should also be considered in the acute therapy of rapid cycling. According to recent investigations by the National Institute of Mental Health, calcium antagonists and, above all, nimodipine may turn out to be a therapeutic alternative. However, there is an urgent need for more research especially in the field of rapid cycling and hence the following algorithm (Fig. 5.**3**) will certainly only be valid for a limited time.

## Depressive Episodes in Bipolar Disorder

**Lithium:** About one-third of the mild to moderate depressive episodes in bipolar disorder appear to respond to lithium monotherapy. Most of the older studies have shown that lithium is significantly superior to placebo in this patient sample. Since, in addition, most patients are on lithium prior to the start of acute treatment, the first logical step in these cases is to check the lithium level and, if necessary, to increase the daily dose.

With regard to antiepileptic agents, alternatives to lithium were rather limited until just recently. Although mild antidepressive efficacy of both carbamazepine and valproate has been reported, there is still a need for large controlled studies. On the other hand, the antidepressive efficacy of lamotrigine in bipolar depressive patients has been demonstrated in a large, placebo-controlled study. A disadvantage of lamotrigine monotherapy is the required slow titration phase so that a rapid onset of the antidepressive action cannot be expected. In combination with a serotonin re-uptake inhibitor, e.g., paroxetine, a more rapid improvement of the depressive symptoms in comparison to an antidepressive monotherapy can be achieved not only for bipolar but also for unipolar depressive patients (Normann et al. 2002).

Finally, one recent investigation has shown that the calcium antagonist nimodipine can be of value for mild depressive states.

**Antidepressants:** With the exception of a few, only mildly depressive patients, the additional administration of an antidepressant is, as a rule, indispensable. However, the above-mentioned comments on the mania-inducing effects of tricyclic antidepressants must be kept in mind. Besides serotonin re-uptake inhibitors (SSRI) and MAO A inhibitors, bupropione – which has noradrenergic and dopaminergic activities – is widely used in the U.S.A. However, this drug has as yet only been approved in several countries for the treatment of nicotine withdrawal symptoms. As far as the antidepressants of the latest generation are concerned, there are as yet only few substantiated data with regard to the risk of switching. A recent study has shown that venlafaxin is associated with a higher risk of switching than an SSRI (in this case paroxetine). Fig. 5.**4** shows a possible treatment algorithm for non-psychotic bipolar depression.

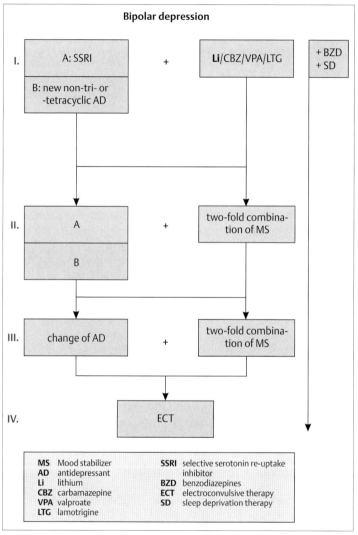

Fig. 5.**4**    Treatment algorithm for depressive episodes in bipolar disorder.

An additional antipsychotic treatment is occasionally also necessary when psychotic features arise or there is a pronounced focusing of thoughts on depressive subjects. Atypical antipsychotic agents should always be preferred in these cases, not only because they may also exert an additional antidepressive efficacy and thus favorably influence the entire course of the illness.

### 5.1.2  Continuation Treatment (Stabilization Phase)

After the acute symptoms have subsided two principle problems remain: the prevention of a direct relapse and, respectively, the switch to the opposite mood state.

This does indeed create some pharmacological difficulties. Classical antipsychotic agents can induce a depressive episode during the subsiding mania; drastic discontinuation attempts, however, may also provoke a recurrence of mania. A similar situation exists in the subsiding depressive phase: on the one hand antidepressants may trigger mania while, on the other hand, their abrupt discontinuation is accompanied by a considerable risk of relapse. Both substance classes, antidepressants and antipsychotics, especially phenothiazines, can also trigger or reinforce rapid cycling.

Accordingly, this time period requires careful reduction of the drug doses with close monitoring of the psychopathology. It is most important in this critical phase to continue the mood stabilizer that was acutely effective in unchanged doses for at least six months with close monitoring of the serum level. This time span is only an approximate guideline; if information about the natural duration of an episode in the absence of medication is available, the mood stabilizer therapy should be continued in unchanged doses for a time clearly exceeding this period.

### 5.1.3  Maintenance Therapy (Prophylaxis)

Maintenance treatment starts after complete remission of the symptoms and the stabilization phase. At present the recommendations are to continue acute treatment for at least one year after a first manic episode. Prophylaxis must be considered at the latest after the second episode and becomes mandatory after the third episode. The Dutch consensus recommendations shown schematically in Fig. 5.**5** represent a good aid as to when prophylaxis should be in-

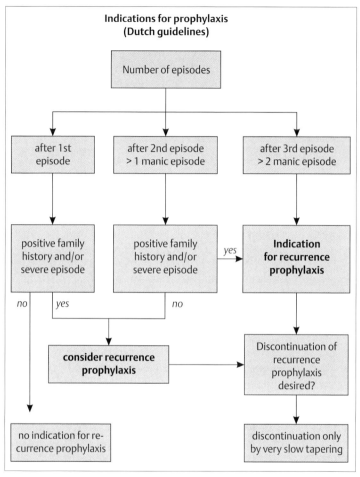

Fig. 5.**5**  Indications for recurrence prophylaxis (Dutch guidelines, after Nolen et al. 1998).

troduced. Provided that the drug is well tolerated, the patient should continue this prophylaxis for the rest of his/her life, keeping in mind that the vulnerability for new episodes usually increases with age.

If the patient should desire to discontinue for acceptable reasons such as planned pregnancy or because of intolerance of the drug, the medication should be reduced very slowly. Abrupt discontinuation, e.g., of lithium, is known to provoke a relapse within a few weeks in up to 50% of the patients.

## 5.2    Non-Pharmacological Treatment Strategies

### 5.2.1  Acute Treatment

**Electroconvulsive therapy (ECT):** As already mentioned in preceding sections, electroconvulsive therapy represents an alternative therapy at various points in the treatment algorithms. The use of ECT is judged differently from country to country. For example, it is used in Germany exclusively for the treatment of refractory illness whereas, for comparison, it is used about 50 times more frequently in Great Britain. The indication for ECT may exist, besides for refractoriness to drug treatment, also for pregnancy which places restrictions on drug treatment and for patients at high risk for suicide in whom a rapid improvement is required, such as, e.g., in mixed mania. In these cases the early use of ECT can be considered, as well as for severe and, especially, psychotic manias and depressions.

A discontinuation of the prior medication is generally only needed for antiepileptic agents and benzodiazepines, in particular when the better tolerated, unipolar stimulation technique is employed. However, for unipolar stimulation over the non-dominant hemisphere there is one report on the deterioration of manic symptoms on. For this reason, bipolar stimulation is often preferred, especially in the U.S.A.

Most studies have demonstrated the superiority of ECT over lithium in the treatment of acute, severe manias. About 80% of the patients benefit from ECT (Prien and Potter 1990).

The success rate for depressive episodes in bipolar disorder is similar. Janicak and co-workers (1985) reported therapeutic success for 78% of the ECT patients as compared to 64% among those treated with tricyclic antidepressants.

However, the risk for a switch from depression to mania is estimated to be about 7%. Furthermore, the rapid therapeutic success of ECT does not, in general, eliminate the need for further drug treatment for prevention of relapses. Even so, there are individual case reports on the successful use of low frequency ECT for prophy-laxis. ECT may possibly also interrupt a rapid cycling course of the disorder.

With regard to side effects, it must be considered that patients taking lithium in addition to receiving ECT in general have a higher risk of a protracted post-ECT confusional state.

**Transcranial magnetic stimulation:** On account of the relatively high technical expenditure of ECT, it is of increasing interest to assess the extent to which repetitive transcranial magnetic stimulation (rTMS) can be used to treat bipolar disorder. There are first studies on its antidepressant efficacy, albeit in mixed collectives of uni- and bipolar depressive patients. Case reports are also indicative of an antimanic activity whereby a right-temporal stimulation seems to be superior to a left-temporal stimulation for mania (and, in con-trast, the left-temporal stimulation may possibly have a stronger antidepressant efficacy).

On the whole, however, this field has not as yet been the subject of much research and a rapid expansion of our knowledge is to be expected in the next few years.

**Sleep deprivation therapy:** Sleep deprivation represents another al-ternative for the acute treatment of depressive episodes. A survey of the literature reveals an average response rate of 59%. However, sleep deprivation is accompanied by a high risk for a switch over to mania; thus the concomitant administration of a mood stabilizer is recommended. Furthermore, the therapeutic response is often only of short duration; the majority of patients experience a depres-sive relapse after the first full night's sleep. This may possibly be al-leviated by a stepwise displacement of the sleeping time after total sleep deprivation in which the patient is kept awake for the second half of the night for several nights in succession – sleep phase ad-vance therapy (Berger et al. 1997).

**Light therapy:** Patients with bipolar I disorder often experience sea-sonally-dependent affective episodes (SAD). A large multicenter study of SAD patients with winter depressions demonstrated a 60–80% success rate of light therapy. Similar to other non-drug modalities, a concomitant mania protection by a mood stabilizer is also necessary.

## 5.2.2 Relapse Prevention

In distinction to acute treatment which, for example, includes ECT as a monotherapy alternative to drug therapy, all non-drug treatment strategies for relapse prevention are to be considered as supplements to the drug-based episode prophylaxis.

Psychotherapy and supporting sociotherapeutic measures may be important in this respect. They have educational character for managing the illness, for stabilizing the patient and his/her family and, last but not least, can increase the adherence to medication.

**Psychotherapeutic strategies:** Topics that are relevant to the treatment of bipolar patients include, among others 1) the handling of the drugs, 2) the recognition and handling of the first signs of relapse into a depressive and/or manic phases, 3) learning to differentiate between personality traits and illness, building or rebuilding functioning social relationships, and 5) learning strategies to deal with stress and burdens of daily life (Meyer and Hautzinger 2000). Cognitive behavioral therapy helps the patient to cope with dysfunctional thoughts and may enhance reliable and compliant use of medication in individual therapy plans. Further individual therapy modalities currently under study include interpersonal psychotherapy (IPT) combined with social rhythm therapy in which the patient should learn to follow a regular daily course of life with avoidance of recurrence risk factors such as lack of sleep.

Group therapy can also lead to success, especially with regard to the stability of family relationships and compliance with treatment plans.

A symptom management program as outlined by Perry et al. (1999) can add additional profit. In this program the patients learn how to recognize early symptoms of their illness and how to react to them, for example, by the early start of an additional drug therapy. Such a procedure has indeed proved to be successful in prophylaxis of mania but not in recurrence prevention of a bipolar depression.

Inclusion of family members in behavioral therapy strategies seems to be particularly important. By this the frequency of rehospitalization can be significantly reduced. Relevant programs such as the BFM-BP [behavioral family management for bipolar disorder, Miklowitz (1996)] are currently most frequently used.

## 5.3 Drugs for the Treatment of Bipolar Affective Disorder

### 5.3.1 Lithium

The administration of lithium salts remains the standard treatment for manic syndromes and for the prophylaxis of bipolar affective disorder. In manic syndromes that are accompanied by high degrees of excitation and delusional symptoms, the additional administration of antipsychotic agents is usually unavoidable. In cases with numerous manic episodes in the previous history, as well as in the presence of atypical symptoms (mixed states, psychotic features) and with rapid cycling, a poorer response to lithium must be expected.

**Dosages:** The therapeutic range for lithium ions is very narrow so that a close monitoring of the serum level is very important. Serum lithium concentrations of less than 0.6 mmol/l increase the risk of a relapse whereas appreciable side effects can occur at a level of 1.2 mmol/l; intoxications are possible at even higher levels.

- Serum lithium concentration for efficacy in mania:
  1.0 – 1.2 mmol/l;
- Serum lithium concentration for a prophylactic effect:
  0.6 – 0.8 mmol/l.

For practical use, a sustained release lithium formulation should be given twice daily. A constant serum level will then be achieved after one week, at which time the first serum level determination should be made.

Lithium is almost completely excreted by the kidneys with a half-life time of between 14 and 30 hours. As a result of the long half-life the effects of dose changes on the steady-state serum level are only noticeable after about 5 days. Furthermore, determinations of the lithium level should be made standardized 12 hours after the last administration, otherwise considerable errors may arise.

Lithium ions are not bound to plasma proteins and are not metabolized. Accordingly, dehydration and a reduction of the glomerular filtration rate may be accompanied by an increase in the lithium plasma level. In cases of hyponatremia lithium absorption is increased with the result that the lithium level increases. Furthermore, it should be noted that some drugs also increase the lithium level, for example, non-steroidal anti-inflammatory drugs (NSAID), calcitonin and ACE inhibitors. Although an increased neurotoxicity has been observed in some cases upon concomitant administration of lithium and an antipsychotic agent (especially haloperidol) – but also with carbamazepine – these drug combinations are generally well tolerated.

**Starting lithium therapy:** Because of the possible occurrence of renal dysfunction as well as hypothyroidism, creatinine clearance and thyroid values should be carefully monitored prior to starting treatment with lithium.

**Control examinations prior to lithium adjustment:**
- Blood count,
- Renal function (serum creatinine and creatinine clearance),
- T3, T4, TSH,
- ECG, EEG,
- Pregnancy test,
- Body weight and neck circumference.

During the first six months of a lithium therapy, kidney and thyroid functions should be checked at 2- to 3-month intervals. Thereafter, these controls may be performed every 6 to 12 months.

**Adverse reactions:** The symptoms of lithium intoxication include vertigo, slurred speech, ataxia, and finally also rigor, hyperreflexia, epileptic seizures, and, in extreme cases, coma. In particular, mild side effects may occur at the start of a lithium therapy and can often lead to patient non-compliance. These include: muscle weakness, tiredness, polypisia, and polyuria as well as a fine tremor. Weight gain as well as concentration and memory impairments may arise after long-term administration of lithium (see Table 5.**3**). The fine tremor can usually be controlled satisfactorily with the β-blocker propranolol (up to $3 \times 4$ mg/day), although this should not be a long-term medication (since it is, among others, depressiogenic).

   Although the responsible physicians often do not pay much attention to these side effects and merely accept them as unavoidable, naturalistic studies have shown that patient compliance must often be judged as very poor just on account of these side effects.

Table 5.**3**   The most important side effects of lithium therapy

| Early side effects | Late side effects |
| --- | --- |
| tiredness | weight gain |
| vertigo | renal dysfunction |
| polyuria and polydipsia | hypothyroidism |
| fine tremor | memory impairments |

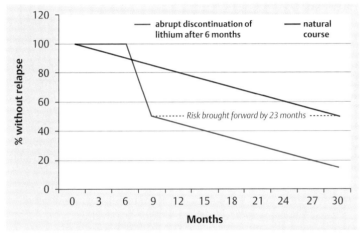

Fig. 5.**6**   Abrupt discontinuation of lithium treatment after 6 months duration leads in 50% of the cases to an immediate relapse. In this way the "natural" course of the illness is de facto brought forward by 23 months (after Goodwin 1994).

Accordingly, the therapeutic success of lithium under naturalistic conditions is disappointing (Gitlin 1995, Maj et al. 1998, Kulhara et al. 1999). Since, however, as already mentioned, the abrupt discontinuation of lithium carries a high risk of a rapid relapse, thus representing a higher danger of suicide, one must consider whether the start of a lithium therapy may put the patient at greater risk as a consequence of doubtful compliance (see Fig. 5.**6**).

If lithium is taken during the first three months of pregnancy, there is possibly an increased risk of congenital abnormalities (mostly cardiovascular malformations). The lithium level is difficult to control in the perinatal period and, after delivery, the children of lithium-treated mothers often exhibit a floppy infant syndrome. Lithium passes into the milk, thus administration of lithium to nursing mothers must also be carefully evaluated.

Absolute contraindications for lithium salts are severe disorders of renal function, as well as cardiovascular diseases. Caution is also required with pre-existing skin diseases (psoriasis) and neurological disorders.

Indispensable prerequisite for lithium prophylaxis is the certainty that the patient will conscientiously take the drug as prescribed and that an uncontrolled discontinuation will not occur. Patients who have taken lithium for 6 months and then abruptly stop it bring forward the risk of relapse by about 23 months in comparison to the natural course (i.e., that of patients who have never taken lithium) as was shown by a study of Goodwin (1994). Furthermore, the opposite side of the medal as far as the anti-suicidal effects of lithium is concerned is that an uncontrolled discontinuation more than triples the suicide risk compared to an untreated patient, i.e., that a rebound suicide tendency is to be feared (Tondo et al. 1998). The hypothesis discussed frequently in the past years on the loss of efficacy of lithium as a result of an intermittent discontinuation, in contrast, has not yet been confirmed in larger studies.

### 5.3.2  Valproate

Similar to lithium salts, valproate exhibits a good efficacy in manic syndromes and probably also as prophylaxis for bipolar affective disorder. The latter assumption is based on numerous open studies. The administration of valproate has the advantage of a rapid onset of action and a very good tolerability. In particular for mixed states, psychotic manias as well as for rapid cycling valproate appears to be even superior to lithium (see Chapter 5.1.1).

**Dosages:** The dosage of valproate for bipolar affective disorder is similar to that for epilepsy. For a manic syndrome, a rapid saturation with up to 20 mg/kg body weight per day is required. Due to its wide therapeutic window, even higher doses are possible in individual

Table 5.**4**   Dosages and plasma levels of valproate

| Mania | Prophylaxis |
| --- | --- |
| Individual high initial dose (20 mg/kg/day) | Individual between about 600 and 2400 mg/day |
| Increase plasma level rapidly to over 50 μg/ml | Plasma level between 50 and 100 μg/ml |

patients. The rapid titration to a serum level of over 50 mg/l appears to be important for a quick antimanic efficacy.

Liquid valproate formulations are useful to achieve a rapid saturation while i.v. formulations are available for patients willing to accept this form of treatment. However, an oral, enteric-coated or sustained release formulation is recommended for long-term treatment. Similar to lithium, a once daily administration is then sufficient (Table 5.**4**).

Valproate has a half-life of about 6–16 hours. The substance is metabolized in the liver and about 90 % is bound to plasma proteins.

The serum levels of substances that are subject to an oxidative metabolism (e.g., phenytoin, lamotrigine, and tricyclic antidepressants) can be slightly elevated by valproate. The serum concentrations of valproate can be lowered by enzyme inducers (such as carbamazepine) and elevated by enzyme inhibitors (such as fluoxetine). Drugs that are also strongly bound to proteins (such as, e.g., acetylsalicylic acid) can displace valproate from the binding sites, resulting in an increase of free valproate and an accompanying intensification of side effects.

**Starting valproate treatment:** Prior to starting a valproate therapy, blood count, hepatic and pancreatic enzymes as well as coagulation parameters must be determined.

With the exception of the treatment of acute mania, the dose of valproate should be slowly increased on account of a possible gastrointestinal intolerance. One can start with about 150 mg/day and then attempt to reach an individual dose of around 600–2400 mg/day. Level determinations are meaningful after about one week with sustained release formulations and serum concentrations between 50 and 100 μg/ml should be reached.

Table 5.**5**    Important side effects of valproate

| Common side effects | Rare side effects |
| --- | --- |
| – Vomiting | – Pancreatitis |
| – Vertigo | – Reversible hair loss |
| – Tremor | – Thrombocytopenia |
| – Asymptomatic increase of liver values | – Polycystic ovary syndrome in young women |
| – Weight gain | – Systemic lupus erythematosus |

The occurrence of asymptomatic increased liver values, leukopenia, or thrombocytopenia is usually not critical but should be followed in every case by close monitoring of laboratory values. In patients who are psychopathologically stable and well adjusted with regard to their doses, serum levels, liver values, and coagulation parameters should be controlled every three months.

**Adverse reactions:** In general, valproate is well tolerated and side effects are thus rather rare. Dose-dependent side effects are gastrointestinal complaints, an asymptomatic elevation of transaminases, and mild neurological symptoms such as tremor or ataxia. An elevation of transaminases is not accompanied by a hepatic dysfunction, is mostly transient, and regresses with dose reduction. A valproate-induced tremor can be treated with propranolol. Above all in long-term therapy, the most significant side effect with a negative impact on compliance is, as with lithium, the gain in weight. Patients with such a predisposition should be reminded in good time to adjust their eating habits accordingly.

Rare side effects are a reversible loss of hair (hair grows again even upon continuation of the therapy) and coagulation disorders. In rare cases the development of a polycystic ovary syndrome and a hyperandrogenism have been observed in young women with epilepsy. Furthermore, to date four cases of a valproate-induced systemic lupus erythematosus have been described (see Table 5.**5**).

In epileptology, valproate-induced fetal liver failure and valproate coma have been described as severe side effects. To date, liver failure has only been observed in children, mostly under 4 years of age, and so it is practically irrelevant for the treatment of adults.

Coma induced by valproate can typically occur in polypharmaco-therapy with other antiepileptic agents, especially barbiturates. However, since one case of valproate coma has already been described for a combination with an atypical antipsychotic agent, the psychiatrist should also be aware of this rare syndrome. Isolated cases of an acute, necrotizing pancreatitis have also been reported so that this possibility should also be considered when there are abdominal complaints.

The administration of valproate in the first trimester of pregnancy increases the risk of neural tube defects. In female epilepsy patients in whom valproate therapy cannot be discontinued, the protective additional administration of folic acid, starting before conception, is recommended. The precursor substance valpromide, commercially available in some countries, e.g., France and Belgium, seems to show a lower teratogenic risk, thus an attempt to change may also be considered. For a detailed discussion on valproate and its use in bipolar disorder, the reader is referred to the German book "Valproat bei manisch-depressiven (bipolaren) Erkrankungen" also published by Georg Thieme Verlag, or to "Anticonvulsants in Mood Disorders" edited by Joffe and Calabrese (Marcel Dekker, New York, Basel, 1994).

### 5.3.3 Carbamazepine and Oxcarbazepine

For many years, oxcarbazepine has also been approved for epilepsy treatment in several countries. Recent studies have demonstrated an antimanic efficacy for oxcarbazepine analogous to that of carbamazepine (Hummel et al. 2002). In the following paragraphs, unless otherwise explicitly stated, all comments about carbamazepine also hold for oxcarbazepine.

Carbamazepine has an efficacy comparable to that of lithium in the treatment of mania; however, mixed states appear to respond better to carbamazepine than to lithium. In such cases, the antimanic efficacy is markedly greater than the antidepressant efficacy in bipolar depression. Carbamazepine in combination with lithium also appears to be superior to lithium monotherapy in cases of rapid cycling.

**Dosages:** The required doses of carbamazepine vary widely from individual to individual; the daily oral dose is usually in the range of

Table 5.**6**    Doses and plasma levels for carbamazepine

| Mania | Prophylaxis |
|---|---|
| Individual high initial dose (600 – 2400 mg/day) | Individual between about 600 and 1800 mg/day |
| Plasma level between 6 and 12 µg/ml | |

600 – 1800 mg (900 – 2400 mg for oxcarbazepine). There are as yet no studies on the relationship between serum levels and clinical efficacy for bipolar disorder. Thus, in general, the optimal plasma level for epilepsy patients is taken as guidance for orientation, which is between 6 and 12 µg/ml (see Table 5.**6**).

As a consequence of an enzyme induction by carbamazepine (but not by oxcarbazepine!) it is able to accelerate its own metabolism. The result is a reduced plasma level after 3 – 4 weeks in spite of a constant oral dose. In addition, it must be remembered that carbamazepine (oxcarbazepine only to a limited extent) can lower the plasma levels of many other drugs such as, for example, antipsychotics, antidepressants, macrolide antibiotics, azoantimycotics, and, in particular, also hormonal contraceptives as well as valproate. Valproate, in turn, can again by elevation of carbamazepine epoxide, an active metabolite, lead to the occurrence of side effects typical for carbamazepine. Calcium antagonists (dilitiazem and verapamil, but not nifedipine and nimodipine) and serotonin re-uptake inhibitors can increase the plasma level of carbamazepine.

**Starting a carbamazepine therapy:** Blood count, liver values and electrolytes must be determined prior to starting a carbamazepine therapy.

With the exception of the treatment of acute mania, the dose of carbamazepine should be increased slowly. In cases of mania, a rapid saturation can be achieved by administration of a carbamazepine suspension (Dose et al. 1991); however, in isolated cases this can lead to vertigo and vomiting as well as mild neurological symptoms (especially double images). In addition, allergic skin reactions have been attributed to rapid dose increases. During the first two months of therapy, blood count, liver values, and electrolytes should be

Table 5.**7**    Important side effects of carbamazepine

| Common side effects | Rare side effects |
|---|---|
| – Vomiting | – Allergic skin reactions |
| – Vertigo | – Aplastic anemia (see text) |
| – Tiredness | – Hyponatremia |
| – Asymptomatic increase of liver values | – Hypocalcemia |
| – Tremor | |

monitored every two weeks; later the interval can be increased to three months.

**Adverse reactions:** Side effects of carbamazepine include an initial tiredness, tremor, allergic skin reactions, and a slight increase in transaminases. The occurrence of aplastic anemia is extremely rare. Mild leukopenia is, however, more common, this is as a rule not critical and does not inevitably progress to aplastic anemia. On account of an activity analogous to that of ADH (antidiuretic hormone), hyponatremia may occur (Table 5.**7**; more frequent with oxcarbazepine than with carbamazepine). In the case of oxcarbazepine, the subjectively impairing side effects such as sedation and vertigo are markedly less severe because this drug is not metabolized to carbamazepine 10,11-epoxide.

The risk of a fetal neural tube defect due to carbamazepine therapy is about 1%. With regard to the nursing period, carbamazepine is considered to be less problematic than lithium or valproate.

The clinical characteristics of antimanic standard treatments with lithium, valproate, and carbamazepine are summarized in Table 5.**8**.

The health-economic importance of a rapid therapeutic success in mania treatment is illustrated in Fig. 5.**7** (after Frye et al. 1996).

### 5.3.4  Lamotrigine

In Europe, lamotrigine (3,5-diamino-6-[2,3-dichlorophenyl]-1,2,4-triazine) was approved for the treatment of epilepsy in the early 1990s and for the prophylactic treatment of bipolar disorder in

Table 5.**8** Lithium, carbamazepine and valproate in mania treatment

| | Lithium | Valproate | Carbamazepine |
|---|---|---|---|
| **Onset of action** | After 5 – 14 days | Within 3 days on rapid saturation | Within one week on rapid saturation |
| **"Loading strategy"** | Poorly tolerated and not without risk | Treatment of choice | Moderately tolerated |
| **Predictors for a better response in comparison to the other substances** | – previous good response<br>– pure euphoric mania in typical bipolar disorder | – previous good response<br>– mixed states<br>– psychotic mania<br>– rapid cycling<br>– co-morbidity | – previous good response<br>– atypical symptoms and courses (similar to valproate) |
| **Predictors for a poorer response in comparison to the other substances** | Atypical symptoms and curses, such as:<br>– mixed state<br>– psychotic mania<br>– rapid cycling<br>– co-morbidity<br>– frequent manias in history (> 10) | – for pure euphoric mania, tendency for inferior efficacy compared with lithium | – for pure euphoric mania, tendency for inferior efficacy compared with lithium |
| **Health-economic aspects** | 40 % longer hospitalization as compared to VPA group (Frye et al. 1996) | 40 % shorter hospitalization as compared to Li and CBZ groups (Frye et al. 1996) | 40 % longer hospitalization as compared to VPA group (Frye et al. 1996) |

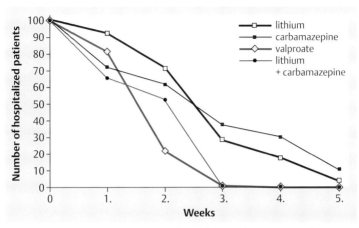

Fig. 5.**7**   Duration of hospitalization depending on the antimanic drug treatment (after Frey et al. 1996).

2003. With regard to interactions with other drugs, the clinical use of lamotrigine is generally uncomplicated (Table 5.**9**). After oral administration lamotrigine is rapidly and completely absorbed and metabolized in the liver with an elimination half-life of about 25 – 30 hours. In general, lamotrigine is well tolerated, the most frequent side effects are headache, occasionally nausea, double images, vertigo or ataxia. About 5 % of the patients may suffer from exanthema at the start of therapy, this side effect depends on the co-medication (above all valproate which inhibits the metabolism of lamotrigine) and the speed of titration. Thus, it is important to follow the slow titration recommended by the manufacturer. In very rare cases, a Steven-Johnson syndrome of allergic origin may arise. Lamotrigine has no influence on the plasma concentration of contraceptives; however, some contraceptives may lower lamotrigine levels. At present, data concerning a possible teratogenic effect are based almost exclusively on epilepsy patients; a markedly lower risk of malformations in comparison to carbamazepine and valproate is currently assumed.

Following several case reports, a first, large open prospective study over 48 weeks has provided indications for efficacy of lamotrigine in 75 bipolar patients of which about one half had rapid cy-

Table 5.**9**  Lamotrigine

| | |
|---|---|
| **Recommended dose** | Start with 25 mg/day in weeks 1 and 2, 50 mg in weeks 3 and 4, 100 mg in weeks 5 and 6, 150 mg in week 7 and 200 mg from week 8 on (recommended dose for anti-depressive and prophylactic treatment). Then individual dose increases up to 500 mg/day are possible. In case of cotherapy with CBZ, the corresponding doses are doubled, with VPA halved. |
| **Possible side effects** | Skin eruptions, in rare cases Lyell syndrome. Rarely tiredness or vertigo. |

cling (Calabrese et al. 1999c). Also about half of the included patients with a depressive phase showed a clear improvement of their symptoms. Furthermore, manic patients also exhibited an improvement; however, the use of lamotrigine in the treatment of mania has proved to be less practicable on account of the slow titration scheme.

Building on these first open studies, in the meantime the efficacy of lamotrigine for the treatment of acute bipolar depressions has also been demonstrated under controlled double-blind conditions (Calabrese 1999). In total, 195 patients were treated over 7 weeks with lamotrigine monotherapy in dosages of 50 or 200 mg or with placebo. On the basis of the Montgomery-Asberg depression scale, it was found that lamotrigine at 200 mg/day achieved a significant improvement in comparison to placebo. A sub-analysis of individual items revealed that, above all, psychic and cognitive symptoms of depression but less the somatic complaints respond to lamotrigine. In this study, a switch to a mania under purely antidepressant monotherapy was not more frequent with lamotrigine than with placebo. Also the discontinuation rates due to adverse events were not different for lamotrigine and placebo. A subsequent open maintenance study showed that the antidepressive effect continued through the observation period of one year. Dosages of up to 450 mg lamotrigine were used in this maintenance study and were well tolerated.

Of particular interest, however, is the prophylactic efficacy of lamotrigine since there is as yet a lack of well-investigated alternatives to lithium. In a randomized, placebo-controlled, double-blind study over 26 weeks, lamotrigine showed efficacy in rapid cycling. 182 patients received either lamotrigine in individual doses between 100 and 500 mg or placebo. The analysis showed that after 26 weeks 41 % of the patients on lamotrigine but only 26 % of the placebo patients completed the study without additional drugs becoming necessary. This treatment success was also reflected in significant improvements in various psychopathological scales such as GAS and CGI-S. Particularly pronounced were the responses of bipolar II rapid cycling patients.

However, not only for rapid cycling patients but also for bipolar patients with a lower episode frequency lamotrigine has shown to exhibit efficacy in the prevention of new episodes in 2 double-blind, controlled studies against lithium and placebo. After an open pretreatment phase with lamotrigine, the patients – after stabilization – were enrolled in these 2 studies lasting 18 months.

In one of the studies, lamotrigine was given in flexible doses between 100 and 400 mg per day, in the other in fixed daily doses of 200 or 400 mg. Lithium was dosed according to the plasma level (between 0.8 and 1.1 mmol/l). In both studies, lamotrigine was significantly superior to placebo with regard to the primary outcome criterion, namely the time to an intervention for a new affective episode and had comparable efficacy as lithium. A differentiated analysis of the results showed in both studies that lamotrigine appeared to be better for protection against depressive episodes while lithium was better for the prevention of manic episodes. In these controlled long-term studies, lamotrigine was also generally well tolerated, only headaches occurred significantly more often with lamotrigine than with placebo.

Of special interest for long-term therapy is the relative weight neutrality of lamotrigine, especially since weight gain represents one of the most frequent reasons for non-compliance and discontinuation of maintenance treatment.

### 5.3.5 Atypical Antipsychotic Agents

The efficacy of typical antipsychotic agents in bipolar disorder, especially in the acute treatment of mania, has been demonstrated by controlled studies and long-term clinical experience. However, their use in high-doses should be limited to the most severe clinical states of mania on account of the well-known and frequent extrapyramidal motor side effects. Accordingly, it was logical to examine the much better tolerated atypical antipsychotic agents for their efficacy in bipolar disorder. Within the group of atypical antipsychotics one can roughly distinguish two subgroups:

The first are drugs that attempt to mimic clozapine in receptor affinity, such as, e.g., olanzapine and in part also quetiapine, while the others are atypical antipsychotic agents that exhibit more a pronounced serotonergic mechanism of action, such as, e.g., risperidone and ziprasidone.

### Clozapine, Olanzapine and Quetiapine

Clozapine as the prototype of atypical antipsychotic agents was first used for bipolar disorder at the end of the 1970s. In small, open studies clozapine exhibited not only a noteworthy antimanic but also an antidepressive and a prophylactic efficacy in otherwise therapy-refractory patients. A wider use of clozapine is limited by the known and potentially severe side effect of agranulocytosis. Accordingly, clozapine was not further investigated for the indication bipolar disorder in methodologically well controlled studies.

There is no such lack of evidence for olanzapine and quetiapine. In particular, olanzapine was examined very early in its clinical development for bipolar disorder in controlled studies. In 2 double-blind, placebo-controlled monotherapy studies, olanzapine was significantly superior to placebo in the treatment of mania (Tohen et al. 1999, Tohen et al. 2000). In these studies the maximum dose was 20 mg per day, however, our present experience and the generally good tolerability of olanzapine allow the use of much higher doses, especially in cases of severe mania. Worthy of special note is that in these studies also patients with mixed states, psychotic symptoms and rapid cycling responded equally well to olanzapine.

In comparison with the clinical standard for mania treatment, valproate, olanzapine proved to exhibit equal efficacy or superiority, respectively, in 2 studies (Zajecka 2003, Tohen 2002). However, the chosen dosages of olanzapine and valproate in the two studies were clearly different. When valproate was administered in an adequate dose so that all patients achieved the established antimanic plasma level, as in the study of Zajecka et al. (2000), an equally good efficacy can be assumed. In a maintenance study over 48 weeks in prolongation of Tohen's trial, there was no significant difference be-

tween olanzapine and valproate with regard to the number of relapses; thus a continuation of olanzapine for maintenance therapy
can indeed be recommended.

In two further studies, olanzapine showed efficacy for episode
prophylaxis against placebo and in direct comparison with lithium
for a period of 1 year. An exact analysis of the data revealed that
olanzapine even appeared to be superior to lithium for the prevention of manic relapses; however, there was no difference with regard to the number of depressive episodes. Hence, olanzapine can
certainly be considered as a therapeutic alternative in the long-
term prophylaxis for patients whose bipolar illness is characterized
mainly by recurring manias. However, further clinical experience in
this aspect should certainly be collected.

The situation with regard to data for quetiapine is equally comprehensive for acute mania. Quetiapine's acute antimanic efficacy
was tested in a study in which quetiapine was compared to placebo
as an additional drug to a mood stabilizer (Sachs et al. 2002) as well
as in 3 double-blind monotherapy studies against placebo, lithium
and haloperidol as comparators. However, for maintenance and
long-term therapy there are at present no valid data. It seems worth
mentioning that quetiapine has also exhibited a good antimanic efficacy and concomitant good tolerability in children and adolescents in a small but placebo-controlled study (DelBello et al.
2002). This patient population is still too little investigated with regard to pharmacotherapy for bipolar disorder.

**Ziprasidone and Risperidone**

Both substances are characterized by a strong affinity for the
5HT2 A receptor and, in addition, ziprasidone also for the 5HT1 A
receptor. In high doses, however, EPMS may occur because of a distinct D2 receptor affinity. The antimanic efficacy of ziprasidone was
demonstrated in a first double-blind, placebo-controlled study of
197 patients (Keck and Ice 2000). Of interest for clinical use is that
ziprasidone (but also olanzapine) is available as an intramuscular
injectable formulation and thus may represent an alternative to
the injectable, highly potent antipsychotic agents for agitated and
psychotic patients.

In the meantime risperidone has exhibited antimanic efficacy in
three placebo-controlled monotherapy studies as well as in add-on

studies to valproate and lithium (Sachs, Grossman et al. 2002, Yatham 2000). With high dosing, the antimanic efficacy was very pronounced in an Indian monotherapy study; however, extrapyramidal motor side effects occurred. These were comparable in nature and frequency to those of the classical, highly potent antipsychotic agents.

The weight gain rather than the extrapyramidal motor side effects constitute more of a problem with clozapine and olanzapine therapy. With these drugs insulin-refractoriness and a limited glucose tolerance may occur. Quetiapine, risperidone and ziprasidone, in contrast, lead only to minimal or no gain in weight. This makes them especially interesting for long-term therapy, however, in contrast to olanzapine, controlled data on their efficacy in prophylaxis are as yet sparse.

### Aripiprazole

To date, the antimanic efficacy of aripiprazole has been examined in 3 controlled studies. In 2 three-week, placebo-controlled studies it exhibited a significant advantage in one whereas in the second it only showed a trend to a higher efficacy. The latter is explained in the study by an extraordinarily high placebo response rate (38%). In a comparative study with haloperidol over 12 weeks, both drugs showed an equal efficacy with a clear advantage concerning side effects for aripiprazole.

### 5.3.6  Combination Therapies

In clinical practice, combination therapies for bipolar disorder are rather the rule than the exception. In a German census (AMÜP Bavaria) in 1998 an average concomitant administration of 2.46 drugs to hospitalized manic patients was determined. An evaluation of seven university hospitals (Stanley Foundation Bipolar Network) showed that bipolar patients on average received concomitantly 4.1 psychotropic drugs. In order to determine the optimal use of mood stabilizers or combinations thereof, a classification into two classes proved to be useful (Ketter and Calabrese 2002). One group of drugs consists of substances that treat mania, hypomania and mixed states; they act "**A**bove baseline" and can be characterized as class **A** mood stabilizers (Table 5.**10**).

Table 5.**10**   Class **A** mood stabilizers

**1.** Mood stabilization from "above"
**2.** Antimanic efficacy without negatively affecting or triggering a depression
– **lithium, carbamazepine, valproate, atypical antipsychotics, ECT**

Table 5.**11**   Class **B** mood stabilizers

**1.** Mood stabilization from "below"
**2.** Antidepressive efficacy without negatively affecting or triggering manic symptoms.
– **Lamotrigine, with limitations lithium, valproate, olanzapine, ECT**

Table 5.**12**   Combinations of class **A** + class **B** mood stabilizers

**1.** valproate + lamotrigine
**2.** lithium + lamotrigine
**3.** Atypicals + lithium
**4.** Atypicals + lamotrigine

The other group rather treats and protects against the depressive phases of bipolar disorder ("**B**elow baseline") and can be designated as class **B** mood stabilizers (Table 5.**11**). This gives rise to rational combinations (Table 5.**12**).

### 5.3.7  Miscellaneous Potentially Useful Drugs for the Treatment of Bipolar Affective Disorder

**Classical antipsychotics:** In clinical practice antipsychotics are often prescribed in addition to mood stabilizers. Although this may be in-dicated for a short time in acute mania, it is often uncritically con-tinued after this phase. Thus, for example, even in U.S.A. more than half of the patients were still taking mostly typical antipsychotics six months after the mania had subsided. Controlled studies have, however, provided contradictory results on prophylactic efficacy, and the danger of tardive dyskinesias and a malignant neuroleptic syndrome limit their long-term use. Their domains are the excited states during manic phases. A further major problem of their use in bipolar affective disorder is the possibility that they may trigger antipsychotic-induced depressions. When the use of classical antipsychotics cannot be avoided, they should as a rule only be administered for a very limited period of time.

**Benzodiazepines:** Benzodiazepines are used as supplementary treatment in mania with the aim of reducing the hyperactivity and inducing sleep. In particular, the use of clonazepam (1 – 2 mg/day), lorazepam (up to 8 mg/day), and diazepam (up to 40 mg/day) is recommended. This is, in the first line, a symptomatic treatment. However, at least clonazepam and lorazepam appear to have their own, albeit low antimanic action. Treatment with these substances should, however, be strictly limited in time due to the risk of addiction. Benzodiazepines exhibit a wide therapeutic range and have a sedative action even at low doses. At very high doses, however, and especially when administered intravenously, the danger of respiratory depression must be taken into account.

**Antidepressants:** Antidepressants should be used as continuation treatment together with mood stabilizers for bipolar depression. However, antidepressants can, in principle, induce a manic episode in bipolar patients (see Chapter 5.1). There are also reports of the induction of rapid cycling and dysphoric mania so that the long-term course of bipolar disorder may become appreciably poorer.

Recent studies have revealed a trend for the risk of triggering mania to be lower with the use of serotonin re-uptake inhibitors, MAO inhibitors and bupropione (which is only approved in Germany for smoking cessation). These modern antidepressants appear also to have a place in the long-term treatment of bipolar patients: they increase the switching risk to mania only slightly, if at all, but markedly protect against depressive relapses. Dosages and duration of treatment are similar to the standards established for unipolar depression. However, for rapid cycling patients with mild depressions lamotrigine should be considered instead of an antidepressant, and otherwise also a more rapid termination of antidepressant use. Of course, this also holds true for patients who have in their history already switched into mania while on antidepressants.

### 5.3.8 Experimental Treatment Strategies

**Topiramate:** Although open studies have indicated not only antimanic but also prophylactic efficacy, controlled studies could not confirm a significant antimanic efficacy for topiramate. Even when it should prove to be not sufficiently potent for antimanic monotherapy, it is still of interest as a well tolerated co-medication. Open studies, for example, suggest an efficacy for bipolar II patients with rapid cycling. A highly appreciated side effect of topiramate is that it leads to in part drastic weight reductions in obese patients. We may assume that topiramate might be able to compensate the weight gains accompanying, for example, lithium, valproate or olanzapine. Topiramate is, in general, well tolerated; sedation, psychomotor slowing, unspecific central nervous side effects (amnesic aphasia, confusion, slowed thinking) and, rarely, temporary paresthesias have been described as the most important adverse effects. There are hardly any serum level interactions with other drugs; the carbamazepine level may be slightly elevated, the valproate level somewhat lowered.

**Calcium antagonists:** Since a disordered intracellular calcium ion homeostasis has been discussed in the pathophysiology of affective disorder (see Chapter 4.3.1), some investigations have been carried out with various calcium antagonists, especially in patients with acute mania. First results have shown an efficacy for the calcium antagonist verapamil.

However, since verapamil can only poorly cross the blood-brain barrier, further studies in the past years have concentrated on the calcium antagonist nimodipine that can penetrate into the CSF. Therapeutic successes have been reported in patients with acute mania, depression, and above all rapid cycling (Pazzaglia et al. 1998); however, large controlled studies must still be carried out. At the moment a sustained release formulation of nimodipine is not available; hence a 4-times daily administration is necessary because of the short half-life (1 – 3 h) (Table 5.**13**).

**Gabapentin:** Some open studies have reported a positive effect of the new antiepileptic agent gabapentin in patients with bipolar affective disorder, both in acute mania and prophylaxis. However, this was not confirmed in a controlled study on mania. In clinical prac-

Table 5.**13**   Calcium antagonists

| *Nimodipine* | Possible dosages: | 120 – 360 mg/day in 4 doses |
|---|---|---|
|  | Possible side effects: | Hypotension |

Table 5.**14**   Gabapentin

| Possible dosages: | 1200 – 3600 mg/day |
|---|---|
| Possible side effects: | Somnolence, ataxia, nausea |

tice, however, gabapentin appears to be valuable as an additional medication for patients with concomitant anxiety disorders or addiction problems. In addition, gabapentin has an analgesic effect that can be usefully employed for patients with co-morbid pain. Combination therapy is generally not problematic since gabapentin has favorable pharmacokinetics and does not influence the metabolism of other psychotropic agents (Table 5.**14**).

### 5.3.9   Predictors of Efficacy

It is difficult to predict the efficacy of drugs in the treatment of the various mood deflections of bipolar disorder. However, some studies have attempted to make predictions at least for the manic phase (see Tables 5.**1**, 5.**2** and 5.**8**).

A frequent finding is that patients with severe mania, dysphoric mania or mania with concomitant substance abuse respond poorly to lithium treatment. For example, about 40% of the patients with bipolar disorder suffer from dysphoric mania and 60 – 70% of these patients do not benefit from lithium therapy. 30 – 50% of the patients with bipolar disorder experience an episode sequence with depression followed by mania. These patients also respond less well to lithium than those with the more common pattern of mania followed by depression. Also, in cases of rapid cycling lithium is less effective than valproate or carbamazepine (see also Chapters 3.4 and 5.4.1).

Finally, there was one more interesting secondary finding in the controlled mania study with valproate, lithium and placebo (Bowden et al. 1994), namely that patients with frequent episodes of mania showed a very poor response to lithium that was not distinguishable from that to placebo. The efficacy of valproate, in contrast, remained constantly good and was independent of the number of previous manias.

## 5.4 Special Treatment Problems

### 5.4.1 Treatment of Rapid Cycling

The treatment of rapid cycling is generally difficult. As already mentioned, the patients usually respond relatively poorly to lithium therapy.

On the other hand, some studies indicate good efficacy for some antiepileptic agents. More recent studies rather prefer valproate over carbamazepine although no direct comparative studies are available. Valproate and carbamazepine both are more effective in the manic phase than in the depressive phase of rapid cycling, whereas lamotrigine rather seems to be effective in preventing depression. On the whole, valproate can thus be considered as the agent of first choice in the treatment of rapid cycling when mania dominates the clinical picture. Especially in cases with frequent depressive episodes lamotrigine should be preferred since its efficacy has been confirmed in a controlled study. For many patients, however, a combination therapy with several mood stabilizers is unavoidable.

If prophylaxis with lamotrigine is unsuccessful, treatment of the depressive phase often requires the use of antidepressants in spite of the possibility for the induction of a manic phase. In such cases, selective serotonin re-uptake inhibitors are the agents of first choice (see Chapter 5.2.2).

In the rare cases of ultra-rapid cycling the calcium antagonist nimodipine may be useful in combination with mood stabilizers.

### 5.4.2 Co-Morbidities with Bipolar Affective Disorder

Bipolar affective disorder is often accompanied by other psychiatric disorders. Various studies have shown that about 30–50% of patients with bipolar disorder also have an alcohol problem. An alcohol addiction in these patients usually results in a poorer prognosis of the bipolar disorder. These patients spend 3–4 times more time in hospital than patients with bipolar disorder but without substance abuse. Besides other, alcohol-related limitations such as lower compliance in taking the prescribed drugs and unstable social surroundings, the alcohol dependence possibly has a direct impact on the biological rhythm possibly triggering bipolar disorder.

As well as alcoholism, the incidence of anxiety disorders is also higher among patients with bipolar disorder. In particular, panic disorder is about twice as frequent in patients with bipolar disorder as compared to those with unipolar depression. In smaller studies, valproate has shown efficacy in panic attacks. If this is not sufficient, treatment with serotonin re-uptake inhibitors is recommended. These substances have the advantage that, on the one hand, they exert a proven efficacy in panic disorder while, on the other hand, the risk of provoking a manic syndrome is lower in comparison to that with tricyclic depressants.

### 5.4.3   Pregnancy and Nursing Period

For women with bipolar disorder, pregnancy is associated with two principle problems. On the one hand, prophylactic drug treatment can involve the risk of damaging the fetus while, on the other hand, the possible termination of the prophylactic treatment increases the probability of a recurrence which in itself may represent a danger to the unborn baby.

The incidence of congenital damage caused by lithium was originally given as 3% for all types of interuterine damage, with the risk of cardiac malformation being particularly high. More recent analyses have not confirmed this extent; even so, the administration of lithium during pregnancy remains a risk. Malformations have also been reported under carbamazepine and valproate therapy with, in particular, neural tube defects being observed in 1–2% of the cases. In epilepsy treatment, the prophylactic administration of folic acid starting prior to conception is recommended for women who wish to have a baby but who cannot terminate their antiepileptic therapy with valproate.

The decision to continue treatment in women with bipolar disorder must certainly be made on an individual basis under close consideration of the case history. In principle, the danger of fetal damage is largest during the first three months of pregnancy. One can thus consider interrupting drug treatment at least for this period.

In every case, however, the prophylactic therapy should be reinstated after the third month of pregnancy or, at the latest, after delivery since the danger of a recurrence is markedly elevated during the postpartal period.

For the new antiepileptic agents and atypical antipsychotic agents there are as yet no reliable numbers but the malformation risk under lamotrigine seems to be smaller than that under the above-mentioned antiepileptic agents.

Breast feeding is not considered to be a problem with carbamazepine therapy. In principle, it is also possible with valproate and lithium therapy so that in exceptional cases a mother's pressing desire in this regard can be respected.

# References

Akiskal, H., O. Pinto: The evolving bipolar spectrum. Prototypes I, II, III, and IV. In: Akiskal, H. (ed.) Bipolarity: Beyond Classic Mania. Philadelphia: W. B. Saunders, 1999: 517 – 534

Alda, M., G. Turecki, P. Grof et al.: Association and linkage studies of CRH and PENK genes in bipolar disorder: a collaborative IGSLI study. Am. J. Med. Genet. 2000; 96: 178 – 181

American Psychiatric Association: Practice guideline for treatment of patients with bipolar disorder. Washington D. C., 1995

Angst, J.: Verlauf unipolarer depressiver, bipolar manisch-depressiver und schizoaffektiver Erkrankungen und Psychosen. Ergebnisse einer prospektiven Studie. Fortschr. Neurol. Psychiat. 1980; 48: 3 – 30

Angst, J., A. Gamma: A new bipolar spectrum concept: a brief review. Bipolar Disorders 2002; 4 (Suppl. 1): 11 – 14

Bauer M., J. Calabrese, D. Dunner et al.: Multisite data reanalysis of the validity of rapid cycling as a course modifier for bipolar disorder in DSM-IV. Amer. J. Psychiat. 1994; 151: 506 – 515

Bauer, M., B. Ahrens: Bipolar disorder. A practical guide to drug treatment. CNS drugs 1996; 6: 35 – 52

Begley, C. E., J. F. Annegers, A. C. Swann et al.: The lifetime cost of bipolar disorder in the US: an estimate for new cases in 1998. Pharmacoeconomics. 2001; 19: 483 – 495

Berger, M., J. Vollmann, F. Hohagen, A. König, H. Lohner, U. Voderholzer, D. Riemann: Sleep deprivation combined with consecutive sleep phase advance as a fast-acting therapy in depression: an open pilot trial in medicated and unmedicated patients. Amer. J. Psychiat. 1997; 154: 870 – 872

Berrettini, W. H., T. N. Ferraro, L. R. Goldin, S. D. Detera-Wadleigh: A linkage study of bipolar illness. Arch. Gen. Psychiat. 1997; 54: 27 – 35

Berridge, M. J., R. F. Irvine: Inositol phosphates and cell signalling. Nature 1989; 341: 197 – 205

Bialer, M., S. I. Johannessen, H. J. Kupferberg, R. H. Levy, P. Loiseau, E. Perucca: Progress report on new antiepileptic drugs: a summary of the third Eilat Conference. Epilepsy Research 1996; 25: 299 – 319

Bowden, C. L., A. M. Brugger, A. C. Swann, J. R. Calabrese et al.: Efficacy of divalproex vs lithium and placebo in the treatment of mania. The Depakote Mania Study Group. JAMA 1994; 271: 918 – 924

Bowden, C. L., J. R. Calabrese, S. L. McElroy, L. Gyulai et al.: A randomized, placebo-controlled 12-month trial of divalproex and lithium in treatment of outpatients with bipolar I disorder. Divalproex Maintenance Study Group. Arch. Gen. Psychiatry 2000; 57: 481–489

Calabrese, J. R., C. L. Bowden, G. S. Sachs, J. A. Ascher et al.: A double-blind placebo-controlled study of lamotrigine monotherapy in outpatients with bipolar I depression. Lamictal 602 Study Group. J. Clin. Psychiatry 1999 a; 60: 79–88

Calabrese, J. R., D. J. Rapport, S. E. Kimmel, M. D. Shelton: Controlled trials in bipolar I depression: focus on switch rates and efficacy. Eur. Neuropsychopharmacol. 1999 b; 9 (Suppl. 4): S109–S112

Calabrese, J. R., C. L. Bowden, S. L. McElroy, J. Cookson, J. Andersen, P. E. Keck et al.: Spectrum of activity of lamotrigine in treatment-refractory bipolar disorder. Am. J. Psychiatry 1999 c; 156: 1019–1023

DelBello, M. P., M. L. Schwiers, H. L. Rosenberg, S. M. Strakowski: A double-blind, randomized, placebo-controlled study of quetiapine as adjunctive treatment for adolescent mania. J. Am. Acad. Child Adolesc. Psychiatry 2002; 41: 1216–1223

DHEW, Medical Practice Project: a state of the science report for the Office of the Assistant secretary for the US Department of Health, Education and Welfare. Policy Research, Baltimore, MD, 1979

Dose, M., D. Bremer, C. Raptis, M. Weber, H. Emrich: Akut antimanische Wirkung von Carbamazepin-Suspension. In: Müller-Oerlinghausen, B., S. Haas, K. Stoll (Hrsg.): Carbamazepin in der Psychiatrie. Stuttgart: Thieme Verlag, 1989: 100–104

Dunner, D., R. Fieve: Clinical factors in lithium carbonate prophylaxis failure. Arch. Gen. Psychiat. 1974; 30: 229–233

Emrich, H., D. von Zerssen, W. Kissling, H.-J. Möller, A. Windorfer: Effect of sodium valproate on mania. The GABA-hypothesis of affective disorders. Arch. Psychiat. Nervenkr. 1980; 229: 1–16

Fieve, R., S. Platman, R. Plutchik: The use of lithium in affective disorders. I. Acute endogenous depression. Amer. J. Psychiat. 1968; 125: 487–491

Frances, A., J. Docherty, D. Kahn (Hrsg.): The Expert Consensus Guideline series. Treatment of Bipolar Disorder. J. Clin. Psychiat. 1996; 57 (Suppl. 12 A)

Frank, E., D. J. Kupfer, C. L. Ehlers, T. H. Monk et al.: Inducing lifestyle regularity in recovering bipolar disorder patients: results from the maintenance therapies in bipolar disorder protocol. Biol. Psychiatry 1997; 41: 1165–1173

Frye, M. A., L. L. Altshuler, M. P. Szuba, N. N. Finch, J. Mintz: The relationship between antimanic agent for treatment of classic or dysphoric mania and length of hospital stay. J. Clin. Psychiatry 1996; 57: 17–21

Gitlin, M. J., J. Swendsen, T. L. Heller, C. Hammen: Relapse and impairment in bipolar disorder. Am. J. Psychiatry 1995; 152: 1635–1640

Goldberg, J. F., M. Harrow: Kindling in bipolar disorders: a longitudinal follow-up study. Biol. Psychiat. 1994; 35: 70 – 72

Goldberg, J. F., M. Harrow, J. E. Whiteside: Risk for bipolar illness in patients initially hospitalized for unipolar depression. Am. J. Psychiatry 2001; 158: 1265 – 1270

Goodwin, F. K., K. R. Jamison: Manic-Depressive Illness. New York: Oxford University Press, 1990

Goodwin, G. M.: Recurrence of mania after lithium withdrawal. Implications for the use of lithium in the treatment of bipolar affective disorder. Br. J. Psychiatry 1994; 164: 149 – 152

Goodwin, G. M., C. L. Bowden, J. R. Calabrese et al.: A meta-analysis of two placebo-controlled 18-month trials of lamotrigine and lithium maintenance in Bipolar I disorder. 2003, in Druck

Grunze, H., J. Walden: Valproat bei manisch-depressiven (bipolaren) Erkrankungen. Stuttgart: Thieme Verlag, 2000

Grunze, H., J. Walden, S. Dittmann, M. Berger, A. Bergmann, P. Bräunig et al.: Psychopharmakotherapie Bipolarer Affektiver Erkrankungen. Nervenarzt 2002; 73: 4 – 17

Grunze, H., S. Kasper, G. Goodwin et al.: The World Federation of Societies of Biological Psychiatry (WFSBP) Guidelines for the Biological Treatment of Bipolar Disorders. Part I: Treatment of Bipolar Depression. World J. Biol. Psychiatry 2002 a; 3: 115 – 124

Grunze, H., S. Kasper, G. Goodwin et al.: The World Federation of Societies of Biological Psychiatry (WFSBP) Guidelines for the Biological Treatment of Bipolar Disorders. Part II: Treatment of Mania. World J Biol Psychiatry 2003; 4: 5 – 13

Hummel, B., J. Walden, R. Stanpfer et al.: Acute antimanic efficacy and safety of oxcarbazepine in an open trial with an on-off-on design. Bipolar Disorders 2002; 4: 412 – 417

Janicak, P. G., J. M. Davis, R. D. Gibbons, S. Ericksen, S. Chang, P. Gallagher: Efficacy of ECT: a meta-analysis. Amer. J. Psychiat. 1985; 142: 297 – 302

Joffe, R. T., J. R. Calabrese (eds.): Anticonvulsants in Mood Disorders. New York, Basel: Marcel Dekker Inc., 1994

Johnstone, E. C., T. J. Crow, C. D. Frith, D. G. Owens: The Northwick Park "functional" psychosis study: diagnosis and treatment response. Lancet 1988; 16: 119 – 125

Kandel, E., J. Schwartz, T. Jessel (eds.): Principles of Neural Science. 3rd. ed. Norwalk: Appleton & Lange, 1991

Keck, P. E., K. Ice: Ziprasidone in acute mania. APA Abstract 2000; NR 224

Keller, M., P. Lavori, J. Kane et al.: Sub-syndromal symptoms in bipolar disorder: a comparison of standard and low serum levels of lithium. Arch. Gen. Psychiat. 1992; 49: 371 – 376

Ketter, T. A., J. R. Calabrese: Stabilization of mood from below versus above baseline in bipolar disorder: A new nomenclature. J. Clin. Psychiatry 2002; 63: 146 – 151

Kulhara, P., D. Basu, S. K. Mattoo, P. Sharan, R. Chopra: Lithium prophylaxis of recurrent bipolar affective disorder: long-term outcome and its psychosocial correlates. J. Affect. Disord. 1999; 54: 87 – 96

Lubrich, B., D. van Calker: Inhibition of the high affinity myo-inositol transport system: a common mechanism of action of antibipolar drugs? Neuropsychopharmacology 1999; 21: 519 – 529

MacKinnon, D. F., K. R. Jamison, J. R. DePaulo: Genetics of manic depressive illness. Annu. Rev. Neurosci. 1997; 20: 355 – 373

Maj, M., R. Pirozzi, L. Magliano, L. Bartoli: Longterm outcome of lithium prophylaxis in bipolar disorder: a 15 year prospective study on 402 patients attending a lithium clinic. Amer. J. Psychiat. 1998; 155: 30 – 35

Meyer, T. D., M. Hautzinger: Bipolare affektive Störungen. In: Hautzinger, M. (ed.): Kognitive Verhaltenstherapie bei psychischen Störungen. Weinheim: Psychologie Verlags-Union, 2000: 40 – 49

Miklowitz, D. J.: Psychotherapy in combination with drug treatment for bipolar disorder. J. Clin. Psychopharmacol. 1996; 16: 56 – 66

Miklowitz, D. J., M. J. Goldstein: Bipolar Disorder: A Family-Focused Treatment Approach. New York: Guilford Press, 1997

Mukherjee, S., A. M. Rosen, G. Caracci, S. Shukla: Persistent tardive dyskinesia in bipolar patients. Arch. Gen. Psychiatry 1986; 43: 342 – 346

Nolen, W., E. A. M. Knoppert-van der Klein, P. F. Bouvy, A. Honig, J.-L. Klompenhouwer, D. P. Ravelli: Richtlijn farmacotherapie bipolaire stoornissen. Amsterdam: Boom, 1998

Normann, C., B. Hummel, L. O. Scharer et al.: Lamotrigine as adjunct to paroxetine in acute depression: a placebo-controlled, double-blind study. J. Clin. Psychiatry 2002; 63: 337 – 344

Pazzaglia, P., R. M. Post, T. A. Ketter, A. M. Callahan et al.: Nimodipine monotherapy and carbamazepine augmentation in patients with refractory recurrent affective illness. J. Clin. Psychopharmacol. 1998; 18: 404 – 413

Perry, A., N. Tarrier, R. Morriss, E. McCarthy et al.: Randomised controlled trial of efficacy of teaching patients with bipolar disorder to identify early symptoms of relapse and obtain treatment. BMJ 1999; 318: 149 – 153

Pfäfflin, M., T. W. May: Kosten von bipolaren Störungen. In: Deutsche Gesellschaft für Bipolare Störungen e. V. (DGBS e. V.) (ed.): Weißbuch Bipolare Störungen in Deutschland. Hamburg: ConferencePoint Verlag, 2002: 111 – 119

Post, R. M., S. R. Weiss, M. Smith et al.: Stress conditioning, and the temporal aspects of affective disorders. Annals New York Academy of Sciences 1995; 771: 677 – 696

Potter, W. Z., T. A. Ketter: Pharmacological issues in the treatment of bipolar disorder: focus on mood-stabilizing compounds. Canad. J. Psychiat. 1993; 38: 51 – 56

Prien, R. F., W. Z. Potter: NIMH workshop report on treatment of bipolar disorder. Psychopharmacol. Bull. 26 (1990) 409 – 427

Sachs, G. S.: Bipolar mood disorder: practical strategies for acute and maintenance phase treatment. J. Clin. Psychopharmacol. 1996; 16: 32 – 47

Sachs, G., J. A. Mullen, N. A. Devine, D. Sweitzer: Quetiapine versus placebo as adjunct to mood stabilizer for the treatment of acute mania. Bipolar Disord. 2002 a; 4 (Suppl. 1): 133

Sachs, G. S., F. Grossman, S. N. Ghaemi et al.: Combination of a mood stabilizer with risperidone or haloperidol for treatment of acute mania: a double-blind, placebo-controlled comparison of efficacy and safety. Am. J. Psychiatry 2002 b; 159: 1146 – 1154

Sass, H., H. Wittchen, M. Zaudig (eds.): Diagnostisches und statistisches Manual psychischer Störungen (DSM IV). Göttingen: Hogrefe, 1996

Scott, J.: Cognitive therapy of affective disorders: a review. J. Affect. Dis. 1996; 37: 1 – 11

Sharma, R., H. Markar: Mortality in affective disorder. J. Affect. Dis. 1994; 31: 91 – 96

Stanton, S. P., P. E. Keck, S. L. McElroy: Treatment of acute mania with gabapentin. Amer. J. Psychiat. 1997; 154: 287

Stoll, A., W. Severus: Mood stabilizers: Shared mechanisms of action at postsynaptic signal-transduction and kindling processes. Harv. Rev. Psychiat. 1996; 4: 77 – 89

Strakowski, S., S. McElroy, P. Keck Jr., S. West: Suicidality among patients with mixed and manic bipolar disorder. Amer. J. Psychiat. 1996; 153: 674 – 676

Swann, A., C. Bowden, D. Morris et al.: Depression during mania: Effect on response to lithium or divalproex. Arch. Gen. Psychiat. 1997; 54: 37 – 42

Tohen, M., T. M. Sanger, S. L. McElroy et al.: Olanzapine versus placebo in the treatment of acute mania. Olanzapine HGEH Study Group. Am. J. Psychiatry 1999; 156: 702 – 709

Tohen, M., T. G. Jacobs, S. L. Grundy et al.: Efficacy of olanzapine in acute bipolar mania: A double-blind, placebo-controlled study. Arch. Gen. Psychiatry 2000; 57: 841 – 849

Tohen, M., R. W. Baker, L. L. Altshuler et al.: Olanzapine versus divalproex in the treatment of acute mania. Am. J. Psychiatry 2002; 159: 1011 – 1017

Turecki, G., P. Grof, P. Cavazzoni et al.: Evidence for a role of phospholipase C-g1 in the pathogenesis of bipolar disorders. Mol. Psychiatry 1998; 3: 534 – 538

van Calker, D., J. Walden (eds.): Valproat in der Psychiatrie. München: Zuckschwerdt Verlag, 1994

Walden, J., H. Grunze, D. Bingmann et al.: Calcium antagonistic effects of carbamazepine as a mechanism of action in neuropsychiatric disorders: studies in calcium dependent model epilepsies. Europ. Neuropsychopharm. 1992; 2: 455 – 462

Walden, J., H. Grunze, H. Olbrich, M. Berger: Bedeutung von Kalziumionen und Kalziumantagonisten bei affektiven Psychosen. Fortschr. Neurol. Psychiat. 1992; 60: 471 – 476

Walden, J., B. Heßlinger: Bedeutung alter und neuer Antiepileptika in der Behandlung psychischer Erkrankungen. Fortschr. Neurol. Psychiat. 1995; 63: 320 – 335

Walden, J., J. Fritze, D. van Calker et al.: A calcium antagonist for the treatment of depressive episodes: single case reports. J. Psychiat. Res. 1995; 29: 71 – 76

Walden, J., H. Grunze, S. Schlösser, M. Berger, A. Bergmann, P. Bräunig, M. Dose, H. M. Emrich, M. Gastpar, W. Greil, H.-J. Möller, R. Uebelhack: Empfehlungen für die Behandlung bipolarer affektiver Störungen. Psychopharmakotherapie (PPT) 1999; 6: 115 – 123

Wehr, T., D. Sack, N. Rosenthal et al.: Rapid cycling affective disorder: contributing factors and treatment responses in 71 patients. Amer. J. Psychiat. 1988; 145: 177 – 184

Weissman, M., R. Bland, G. Canino et al.: Cross-national epidemiology of major depression and bipolar disorder. J. Amer. med. Assn. 1996; 276: 293 – 299

West, S. A., S. M. Strakowski, K. W. Sax, S. E. McElroy et al.: Phenomenology and comorbidity of adolescents hospitalized for the treatment of acute mania. Biol. Psychiatry 1996; 39: 458 – 460

Williams, R. S. B., L. Cheng, A. W. Mudge, A. J. Harwood: A common mechanism of action for three mood stabilizing drugs. Nature 2002; 417: 292 – 295

Winokur, G., W. Coryell, M. Keller et al.: A prospective follow-up of patients with bipolar and primary unipolar affective disorder. Arch. Gen. Psychiat. 1993; 50: 457 – 465

Wyatt, R., I. Henter: An economic evaluation of manic-depressive illness. Soc. Psychiat. Epidemiol. 1995; 30: 213 – 219

Zajecka, J. M., R. H. Weisler, A. C. Swann: Divalproex sodium versus olanzapine for the treatment of mania in bipolar disorder. American College of Neuropsychopharmacology Annual Meeting Poster Abstracts, 2000

# Index